Timothy Welch, a former dean at Cabrillo College in California, has organized many seminars and conferences, including the Cabrillo Fitness Adventure in collaboration with Dr. Sherman Karpen. He has also managed several arts enterprises, including the Cabrillo Music Festival, the Cabrillo Summer Theatre, the Cabrillo Summer Music Academy, and is founder and director of Cabrillo Suspense Writers Conference. He is the author of two suspense novels entitled *The Tennis Murders* and *The Pro-Am Murders.*

Timothy Welch

TAPE IT OFF!

LOSE WEIGHT QUICKLY AND ENJOYABLY THROUGH SELF-HYPNOSIS

A SPECTRUM BOOK

Prentice-Hall, Inc., Englewood Cliffs, New Jersey 07632

Library of Congress Cataloging in Publication Data
Welch, Timothy L.
Tape it off!
Includes index.
"A Spectrum Book."
1. Reducing diets—Psychological aspects. 2. Autogenic training. I. Title.
RM222.2.W34 1984 613.2'5 83-22892
ISBN 0-13-884635-9 (c.)

Cover design: Hal Siegel
Manufacturing: Pat Mahoney
Editorial/production supervision: Fred Dahl

This book is available at a special discount when ordered in bulk quantities. Contact Prentice-Hall, Inc., General Publishing Division, Special Sales, Englewood Cliffs, N.J. 07632.

A SPECTRUM BOOK

1 2 3 4 5 6 7 8 9 10

Printed in the United States of America

ISBN 0-13-884635-9

PRENTICE-HALL INTERNATIONAL, INC., *London*
PRENTICE-HALL OF AUSTRALIA PTY. LIMITED, *Sydney*
PRENTICE-HALL CANADA INC., *Toronto*
PRENTICE-HALL OF INDIA PRIVATE LIMITED, *New Delhi*
PRENTICE-HALL OF JAPAN, INC., *Tokyo*
PRENTICE-HALL OF SOUTHEAST ASIA PTE. LTD., *Singapore*
WHITEHALL BOOKS LIMITED, *Wellington, New Zealand*
EDITORA PRENTICE-HALL DO BRASIL LTDA., *Rio de Janeiro*

For Jacque, and Tim,
and Nicci, and Dominie,
and Susan—
a trim life!

CONTENTS

FOREWORD

The techniques employed in *TAPE IT OFF!* to modify attitudes and habits in using food and drink are rooted in the research and clinical practice of Stunkard, Mahoney, Hartland, Kroger and Fezler, the Birds, and others and have proven effective with countless patients.

Associating positive images and sensory experiences with good eating and drinking practices, while in the deeply relaxed and concentrated state called self-hypnosis, is the powerful new tool Dr. Welch describes well in this work. The use of a tape recorder with the subject's own voice giving directions is especially appealing and effective.

As with any treatment, users of this book are strongly advised to consult their personal physicians before commencing a weight-loss program. People with a potential for anorexia or bulimia should avoid this procedure.

This technique, used daily, will result in your being able to enjoy *both* the eating experience and the experience of your conscience *after* eating.

Sherman A. Karpen, M.D.

PREFACE

Another "diet book"?

Let's face it: the remission rate for nearly every form of cancer is better than the success rate experienced by people trying to lose weight. Only five percent of dieters who are weighed 12 months later have sustained the loss from their "diets."

Diets don't work.

Changing your attitudes and your self-images, on the other hand, works *very well.*

You can't keep weight off even with "successful" diets because you can't count on a lifetime—or even a few months!—of rigid self-control, with feelings of denial, self-pity, and depression as you regard years and years ahead with no coconut cream pie, or whatever your bête noire.

Slim people are not rigidly controlling their eating behavior. You know that from a lifetime of watching slim people eating what they want while you tell the dinner group that you can't have some desirable dish or other because you're "on a diet!"

The attitude of slim people toward food and drink is different from the attitude held by fat people. It's that simple. They expect much less from food.

Self-hypnosis is the best way to create the new attitudes that will alter your eating habits and, as a by-product and almost an afterthought, allow you to lose weight quickly and with no perception of struggle or self-denial. You will eat less, and you will eat the right foods, and you will enjoy the process. You will put eating and drinking back in their proper places in life: something that you do as an adjunct to living, but not life's main activity.

You will do this by recording a fifteen-minute cassette tape, highly personalized to your specific eating problems, and playing this back to yourself before dinner each night to relax yourself, to invigorate your evening, and to build the new positive attitudes you need for a lifetime of fitness and good weight.

This book will provide you with the "scripts" for inducing the deeply relaxed hypnotic state needed for post-hypnotic suggestion to succeed, and the "post-hyp" scripts necessary to change your attitudes about, and responses to, food and drink.

The techniques described in this book have worked for me personally, trimming 40 pounds in an unstressful way, and so my relationship to the techniques is that of the grateful user. My doctoral degree is not in nutrition.

I acknowledge with gratitude here the work of several weight control research pioneers in behavior modification, including Albert J. Stunkard, Richard B. Stuart and Barbara Davis, John Hartland, William S. Kroger and William D. Fezler, and Vincent Antonetti. Several of the standard structured images devised by Kroger and Fezler have been paraphrased herein and used by permission, as has their double-bind induction technique.* Antonetti's computations for weight-loss rates at various energy levels form the basis for tables in the Appendix. Though the work of many formed the basis for the techniques in this book, responsibility for its depiction remains my own. Keen thanks are due Karen Darneille and Carol Shrum for their tireless transcription and typing of the manuscript.

Finally, in the galaxy of "diet books," this is the only book to show you induction, deepening, and post-hypnotic "scripts" that are specific to individual weight problems. That's why this book is badly needed by an estimated 70 million Americans. If you've read this far, you, too, probably need to TAPE IT OFF!

And you can, you can!

*From *Hypnosis and Behavior Modification: Imagery Conditioning,* by William S. Kroger and William D. Fezler (Lippincott: 1976).

CHAPTER ONE

SELF-HYPNOSIS WORKS!

You're too fat!

Almost everyone in America thinks he/she has a weight problem, and unfortunately, almost everyone is right. We live in a society that eats too much, drinks too much, and sits too much. We have electric can openers, electric letter openers, and electric window openers on our cars. Talking is the most strenuous exercise most of us engage in.

Do you know how long you'd have to talk to lose ten pounds? Don't even think about it . . .

This is a short book designed to be used. You've read other "weight books" before and you've tried "diets" before, so we won't pad the text telling you things you already know—calories do count, only one or two percent of overweight people have glandular problems, you should consult your physician before attempting to lose a large amount of weight, and nutritional balance is important.

This is a "radical" weight program only in two respects: it works, and it gangs together two powerful techniques—hypnosis and behavior modification. It does not contain magic purple sticks and it does not destroy your health. Hypnotism is a safe, widely-used way of dealing with compulsive behaviors. There is no danger of sinking into some sort of "trance pit," nor of harming yourself. This is a positive, humanistic way of supporting your good impulses—not some screenwriter's notion of Svengali manipulating a helpless victim. Hypnosis works—for you.

FAT IS A KILLER

Heart and blood vessel diseases take at least one million lives a year in the United States, where seventy million people are overweight.

Fat is a killer in the sense that it places an extra burden on the heart and other organ systems of the body to carry and service a body that is 20 or 30 or 40 percent over its designed capacity.

But fat is a killer in an even more literal and dangerous sense. Cholesterol, one type of fat, is a major part of the atherosclerotic deposits that clog arteries and cause heart attacks. Saturated fats are found in great quantities in beef, pork, cheese, and other animal foods, and the cholesterol in eggs and meats raises the cholesterol floating around in the body's blood vessels. Many experts believe this is where atherosclerosis starts.

Nutritional research in the past decade has suggested that we should all be eating foods which contain "polyunsaturated" fats of the kind found in fish and many vegetable oils in order to lower blood cholesterol levels. People in Japan eat mainly food that contains a very low saturated fat level. They eat foods containing low saturated fats and high polyunsaturated fats. They also have a decidedly lower rate of heart disease than do Americans.

Even more important, however, is the type of cholesterol present in the blood stream. Recent studies have shown that people with a high ratio of high density lipoproteins to low density lipoproteins have a low risk of coronaries.

There is further evidence that fats may be a cause of colon cancer, and experts on animals have shown that a diet high in fat increases the risk of breast cancer. Caucasian women secrete almost three times the prolactin than do Chinese women, who have a low incidence of breast cancer. Vegetarians, on the other hand, suffer one-half the heart attack deaths that other Americans do, have far lower death rates from breast and colon cancer, and live longer. Unfortunately, eating nothing but vegetables produces a lack of protein and the necessary amino acids the body requires.

All of this is to remind you of what you already know: fat is dangerous for you, and you should get it off. We're going to show you how to do that!

CAN 70,000,000 OBESE AMERICANS BE RIGHT?

You're fat, and you've got company!

With overweight people constituting almost one-third of the total American population, it might be considered that a group of people approaching a majority of the population might be right; maybe fat is okay.

But you know yourself that it isn't; you get tired too easily, you get injured too easily, and you don't get those admiring glances.

Furthermore, counterrevolution is well under way. Jogging has become nearly epidemic; sales of sports shoes are reaching $1 billion per year. Americans also spend $5 billion on health foods and vitamins, $15 billion for diet and exercise books, $1 billion on cosmetic surgery, $6 billion for diet drinks, and $240 million for barbells and aerobic dance programs. Added to this is another $5 billion for expenditures for health clubs and corporation fitness centers, another $8 billion for sporting goods and sportswear, and $1 billion annually for bicycles.

A nearly new field of medicine—sports medicine—now accounts for about $2 billion a year in expenditures, an estimated thirty million runners are jogging throughout the United States, and thirteen million weight lifters are working out in about five thousand health clubs in the United States.

So you're in good company. You're overweight and out of shape, and you're fighting back!

You're fat because you eat and drink too much and because you exercise too little. You eat and drink for a wide variety of reasons besides hunger—remember hunger, that rarely felt pang in the stomach? You're using food and drink for purposes never intended.

And we're going to change all that!

Remember: no pills on this diet . . . no hunger pains . . . no counting of calories . . .

A SHORT HISTORY OF HYPNOSIS

The idea of healing while in a trance state is one of the most ancient of the medical arts, practiced by primitive man who believed that the trance state and the cures obtained in it were religious in origin. Many of the ancient Greek and Egyptian "dream incubation centers"—such as the Temple of Esculapius at Epidaurus—specialized in the dreams that were in all probability induced by what we today would call hypnosis.

The Swiss physician Paracelsus (1493–1541) laid the foundation for the idea that was to come of hypnosis as "animal magnetism" because of his belief that the magnetic nature of stars influenced human beings, and that all magnets in fact influence the human body by means of invisible emanations. Van Helmont (1577–1644) was the first to suggest that a kind of animal magnetism with a potential to influence the minds and bodies of other people could come from the human body. From this belief in "animal magnetism" came the technique of the "laying on of hands" as a means of healing through faith, though latter-day faith healers ascribe its power to God rather than to "magnetism."

The most famous of all the magnetic healers was the Austrian physician Franz Mesmer, who in 1765 passed his medical examination and submitted a thesis based upon the influence of the planets on human health. Mesmer used an elaborate ceremony that was very similar to those employed at the miraculous shrines where the laying on of hands took place. The patient was brought into a dark hall where the windows were thickly curtained and soft music played. The patient was required to be absolutely silent. In the beginning, Mesmer used a large open tub filled with water, iron filings, and powdered glass. At the proper moment, the great magnetist would appear, holding a long iron wand, and pass his hand over the bodies of the patients or touch them with his iron wand. Later in his career, Mesmer dispensed with the iron wand.

Mesmer was successful in curing many people whom other physicians had given up as incurable, and his fame spread. However, the opinion of the established medical profession became increasingly hostile, and in 1784, Louis XVI appointed a Commission to investigate Mesmerism, whose membership included the famous chemist Lavoisier, Benjamin Franklin (the American ambassador to France), and Dr. Guillotine (inventor of the execution device).

The Commission failed to discover any concrete evidence of

"animal magnetism" and concluded that any benefits within the patients were entirely subjective (!).

Today, the curing of illness by subjective means is preferred to that of the scalpel!

Hypnotism was forgotten until 1841, when James Braid, a well known Manchester surgeon, saw the French magnetizer La Fontaine apparently put a girl into a trance. Braid's initial anger gave way to astonishment and interest when he challenged the induction, and he began a series of experiments of his own. He used the trance for medical and surgical purposes and reported good results, as did the English surgeon John Elliotson, a man with a reputation as a "radical" and firebrand for such practices as being one of the first men in the British Isles to use a stethoscope, which had been invented on the continent.

About the same time a Scottish surgeon practicing in India, James Esdaile (1808–1859), began to use hypnosis to control surgical pain, and over a 5-year period performed over three hundred major surgical procedures using only hypnosis as an anesthetic. The majority of these operations involved removing massive tumors of the scrotum; nineteen were limb amputations. The mortality rates for removal of these tumors dropped from 50 percent to 5 percent, but medical journals refused to publish his results. Probably one reason hypnosis as an anesthetic did not gain wider use at this time was the parallel development of chemical anesthetics (nitrous oxide in 1844, ether in 1846, and chloroform in 1847). Chemical agents were easier and quicker to administer, even though they were more dangerous.

In this century, Clark Hull (1884–1952) and Ernest Hilgard have been principal investigators into the process of hypnosis. Hilgard is till active at the Stanford University Laboratory of Hypnotic Research.

In 1955, the British Medical Society officially recognized hypnosis as an accepted medical tool; the American Medical Association followed in 1958. Certifying boards were set up in 1960.

The use of hypnosis has come from ancient origins through a period of mysticism and charlatanism, and has emerged into a widely used, effective medical tool today.

You are going to discover its effectiveness for yourself!

HYPNOSIS, BEHAVIOR MODIFICATION, AND WEIGHT CONTROL

Learning theory—how people come to think what they think—teaches us that overeating and eating the wrong foods are learned.

All those snack foods you crammed into your mouth were foods you *learned* to eat.

The carrots were always in the store, but you learned to get the cupcakes. Or the doughnuts.

You *learned* to do this.

The "unlearning" of this kind of response has come to be called "behavior modification," a chunky kind of phrase to describe what has been the most effective weight loss technique devised until the clinical technique presented in this book—wedding the power of hypnosis to the long-term effectiveness of "behavior mod."

Conditioning, through covert sensitization and desensitization, has been widely effective in clinical practice. They are two sides to the same coin. Using desensitization, a patient loses his anxiety over, say, flying or public speaking, through repeated pairings of pleasant experiences with the feared experience, until the fear reaction is "extinguished." With sensitization, just the opposite takes place as a patient with too great a love of ice cream continually compares the idea of that ice cream with his recollection of a personal experience of nausea.

Best of all, studies and clinical practice have found that the conditioning of these responses under hypnosis has been more durable, quicker, and less likely to extinguish.

In other words, by using the powerful focusing and relaxing qualities of hypnosis, and the relearning techniques of behavior modification, you can rebuild your responses to anxiety and depression so that better kinds of behavior result.

You don't *have* to reach for the refrigerator door when the washing machine breaks down at the same time that your car's transmission drops onto the highway and your son's "F" in algebra turns out to be generosity on the part of the teacher.

You can change!

In the future, we are going to see a variety of superb new "obesity technologies" put in place by the advances of scientific knowledge: control of brain hormones, such as cholecystokinin that control appetite and digestion; and "calorie-free" foods whose tastes and flavors are indistinguishable from those they replace, such as Procter and Gamble's synthetic fat substitute, sucrose polyester, which is not absorbed in the intestine.

But these technologies remain in the future, and for the present and foreseeable future, your best bet is to

TAPE IT OFF!

RELAXATION AND SELF-HYPNOSIS

Anxiety is a root cause of many kinds of emotional turmoil resulting in a variety of destructive kinds of behavior, such as overeating, chain smoking, and depression, and resulting in a vast number of health disorders such as ulcers, asthma, hypertension, and certain kinds of heart disease.

A key part of your change will be in learning to produce a response of relaxation to stressful events in life. Self-hypnosis, transcendental meditation, Zen, and yoga are all self-induced states and share many similarities:

- fixing your attention on an external object or mental image
- developing a passive attitude and ignoring the immediate environment
- using a quiet, non-distracting setting

Self-hypnosis alone, practiced fifteen minutes per day with no post-hypnotic script, would improve your state of anxiety, and hence help to remove the cause of your overeating.

But when you pair self-hypnosis with the imaging and covert sensitization of behavior mod, you are sure to change your eating and drinking habits and—almost as a side effect—lose that unwanted weight!

So, take fifteen minutes per day, relax, and *TAPE IT OFF!*

CHAPTER TWO

DOING IT RIGHT!

You've seen advertised in magazines and in newspapers plenty of cassette tapes that claim to help you stop smoking, reduce phobias, and to lose weight.

The idea of using cassette tapes in a self-suggestion way is a widely used technique today.

Besides health issues, tapes are available for self-improvement, financial, and investment areas as well; they're based on the same psychological foundations that we speak about in this book—that you can give yourself effective, powerful advice!

WHY MAKE YOUR OWN?

Since many cassettes are available on the market, you might ask yourself why you should go to the trouble of making your own, highly personalized tape? After all, why not just go down to the store and buy one or check a tear-out coupon from a magazine?

Because you want to *do it right!*

For the techniques of behavior modification to work, you must write into your own "script" very specific "cues" (in psychologist language) that will act to change your habits. For example, if you are addicted to a particular brand of peanut butter, you must picture that specific label, its colors and shape. If you eat too many ice cream sundaes while sitting in a particular chair watching a particular television show, you must picture these events specifically.

Obviously, no pre-recorded tapes that are sold on a mass basis can be this personal, and consequently cannot be as effective. You would only need to spend a few minutes writing your script and recording it—and the rest of your life enjoying its benefits!

UPDATING YOUR TAPE

You will want to rewrite your script every few months to keep pace with the changing you.

When the advice you are giving yourself while under hypnosis takes hold and changes your behavior, you will want to focus on other problem behaviors that need to be improved.

Most people arrive at an obese state through a group of problem behaviors and not just one. On the other hand, if you try to "load up" your script with all your problem behaviors at one time, you may find that you are trying to change too many things all at once.

For this reason it's a good idea to list all of the things you do—and the things you *don't* do—that cause you to be fat. Then choose three or four of them for one script, and three or four more for the next script, and so on. When you see your behaviors have changed, simply retape your script and begin a new series of changes in yourself.

Remember, you know exactly what the problems are better than anyone else. With the help of the techniques in *TAPE IT OFF!* you can make these corrections in your behavior!

You are like a sailboat out on the ocean: You're drifting off course, and you need to give yourself a few instructions on trimming sail to change the course of your life.

EQUIPMENT YOU WILL NEED

Luckily, the "hardware" you will need to tape your own autohypnosis tape is widely available and inexpensive.

A variety of cassette tape recorders is on the market priced from $25 on up, and the tape feature is commonly incorporated in many high fidelity systems. However, I'd suggest buying an inexpensive, small unit that you can leave in your bedroom or another quiet place, close at hand.

Since these tapes last about 15 minutes, you will need a cassette of at least that length to record your script *on one side*. (Obviously, you do not want to wake yourself out of your trance-state to turn over the cassette!)

One feature is highly desirable on your cassette recorder: An ear piece that goes from the recorder into your ear so that the message is private and personal. These ear pieces are commonly sold with tape recorders as part of the equipment, so they are readily available for your use.

Remember, you are going to be giving yourself some very candid and frank advice about matters that are very personal to you, and it will inhibit your ability to relax fully into a trance-state if your tape recording is blaring out into the public airwaves for family or neighbors to overhear!

THE RELAXATION ENVIRONMENT

You are going to need a place where you can relax every day for about fifteen minutes with little fear of being interrupted—ideally, just before the evening meal preparation or the dining or cocktail hour.

For most people, a bedroom is the answer, particularly if the door can be locked or blocked with a chair to prevent sudden, noisy entrances by children. You should lie on your bed, with a comfortable pillow, with your tape recorder by your side. Take your shoes off and wear loose clothing. Remove glasses or contact lenses. Close the curtains, and if there is a phone in the bedroom that can be unplugged, do so. *You want to be relaxed, comfortable, and undisturbed for this fifteen minutes.* Afterwards you will feel full of energy!

Why all this care about privacy and a locked door? You may gain the feeling that you are doing something potentially dangerous.

Not at all.

There is no damage you will sustain by being interrupted from your trance-state before you have completed listening to your tape. But it will "waste" that particular learning period, and will lengthen the time it takes you to change your eating ways. It may make you feel slightly irritable, thereby increasing your likelihood of poor behavior in the kitchen.

Many people simply tell children that they're going to take a little nap before dinner; in effect that is exactly what you will be doing: taking the deepest and most highly refreshing nap you have ever experienced, while giving yourself excellent advice!

You are going to *love* your daily fiften minute "nap"!

YOUR MASTER'S VOICE

The fact that you are recording your own tape in your own voice and way of speaking is important to changing your behavior.

At first when you hear yourself speaking, your voice will seem strange or unnatural to your ears, but this will soon pass. Very quickly you will realize that you are listening to the one person who knows how you feel, the voice of the one person you can't fool, and the one person most sympathetic to you—the voice of reality.

USING INDUCTION AND "POST-HYP" SCRIPTS

Induction scripts, as you might expect, are used to put you into a deeply relaxed and receptive trance-state. You are "hypnotized" by using the induction script.

If this book teaches you no other thing than the ability to deeply relax yourself and remove your anxieties on a daily basis, it will have served a marvelous function. For most people, anxiety and fretting—quite often over events they cannot control or hope to influence—represents the biggest reason that they eat too much of the wrong foods. Using the induction script and deeply relaxing yourself before the evening meal on a daily basis will produce excellent and positive changes in your life.

However, when you also write your own post-hyp script (a script that makes strong suggestions to you about changing problem behavior), you have the most powerful weapon available in the fight against fat!

The post-hyp script that you will write and record on your tape will focus on the particular problems that you as an individual have, and will help you change the way you are dealing with that problem—overeating.

Beginning in Chapter 8 are several post-hyp scripts dealing with common abuses of food and the reasons for those abuses. You can use these post-hyp scripts as a basis to write your own, very particular script that focuses on your own area of improvement. You will be shown exactly how to do this in Chapter Eighteen.

For your first script it is perfectly legitimate to "cut and paste" applicable ideas from these post-hyp scripts, and then simply add sentences and phrases that make it specific for you. As you gain more confidence in your ability to write post-hyp scripts and to give yourself guidance, you may write your own post-hyp scripts from scratch.

The main thing you should remember is this: By taking charge and making your own tape, you are taking charge of your own life to change it in a positive way. The technique absolutely works! You will bring your weight to its proper level, you will relax more while you are living your life, and you will enjoy your life more!

(As with any weight-loss program, you should consult your physician before beginning to drop that poundage.)

Now let's see how to put yourself into a deeply relaxed trance-state . . .

CHAPTER THREE

EYE FIXATION AND ARM LEVITATION

Self-hypnosis is, first of all, deep relaxation, with attention focused in a very narrow circle on a particular message you are giving yourself. This state of deep relaxation shares many of the physical benefits that you find in yoga, zen techniques, transcendental meditation, the relaxation response, and many other techniques for producing very real, measurable health benefits. Some of these have lessened the likelihood of high blood pressure and all its family of diseases.

The idea of an induction script, then, is to produce this deep and marvelous sense of relaxation. If *TAPE IT OFF!* were to give you no other benefit than this technique of deep and energizing relaxation, you would feel well satisfied. But we're going to change your state of mind about eating and drinking, too, and you are going to lose some weight!

The following induction scripts are printed in the order you should try them, and provide some variety in the ways you will enter the deeply relaxed state. Once you become practiced in them, you can use a "take-out" from one of them to relax yourself at stressful, food-abusing times.

Start with this technique first: eye fixation, arm levitation.

Read in a low, soft voice in a monotone.

You will look at a spot directly above your head on the ceiling . . .

Pick a spot on the ceiling just above your hairline; keep staring at it . . .

As you stare at it, the first sensation you'll learn how to control is that of heaviness . . .

Your eyelids are getting very . . . very . . . heavy . . .

They are getting heavier . . . and heavier . . .

Your eyes are beginning to blink . . .

Your eyes are blinking and you've just swallowed . . .

This is a good sign that you're getting more and more relaxed, and now, at the count of three, if you really wish to gain mastery and control over your weight, you'll first learn to control the closing of your lids . . .

The feeling of heaviness in your eyelids by this point will be pronounced, and you will want to close them quickly. Try to control the speed of closing your eyes, as this will relax you more deeply.

At this point, you'll notice that you want to close your lids because they're getting very . . . very . . . tired . . .

Promptly, precisely, and exactly, you will close your lids . . . not because you have to, but because you really want to . . .

Don't close your eyelids too rapidly, but close them gently . . . At the count of three your lids are closing tighter and tighter together . . .

You will really feel that tightness . . .

One . . . two . . . three . . .

Good . . .

Feel that tightness . . . glued together . . .

Now let the eyeballs roll up into the back of your head . . .

Now let them roll back down into their regular position . . .

As they return to their normal position you will notice that your lids are stuck even tighter and tighter together . . .

Once again, the feeling of the eyelids being glued together so they cannot be opened is a strong one, and shows you that you can control the actions of your own body by conscious suggestion. You will be able to control your appetite and your response to the kinds of food you eat, too!

Now you will imagine that your entire body . . . from your head to your toes . . . is becoming very . . . very . . . relaxed . . .

You can relax more deeply by picturing a very relaxing situation . . . a memory of a very relaxing time . . .

The point here is to spend a moment remembering one of the most deeply relaxing experiences that you can recall. It might be a warm bath. It might be a massage. It might be the aftermath of sex. The point is to remember it and to picture in detail the physical environment in which it took place: the feeling of the porcelain, the texture of the carpet, or the smells, the color of the light . . . all of these and more detail will make the experience more vivid to you and relax you more deeply.

Remember: *we have used the example here of a soothing, warm, bath, but in writing your own script in Chapter 18 you should insert whatever your own personal experience of a deeply relaxing time has been.*

Remember yourself taking a soothing, warm bath . . .

You are relaxing deeper and deeper . . .

You can feel the hot water and see the steam rise, and as you see these things, the deeper into relaxation you will go . . .

The more vividly you can see yourself in the tub . . .

See the sliding glass doors . . .

See the soap dish . . .

The more deeply relaxed you'll be . . .

The details like the two that follow are crucial to deepening your relaxation!

Feel the hot water coming up to your armpits . . .

Hear the sound of the water from the faucets . . .

The more deeply relaxed you will be . . .

You are doing fine . . .

Your breathing is getting slower . . . deeper . . . and more regular . . .

Now, if you really wish to go deeper, to gain more mastery over yourself, and to control your eating and your drinking habits, you must next learn how to raise your arm in a controlled manner . . .

Listen very carefully to these instructions and carry them out to the best of your ability . . .

The truth of this particular statement will be demonstrated to you shortly. Notice how easily your arm lifts up—more easily than you could raise it in a conscious way. You are also able to keep that arm up for a much longer period of time than you would otherwise be able to do.

This is the technique that stage hypnotists have used for years, in which they are able to get a person's body rigid enough to span the distance between two chairs, allowing people to walk over them as though on a bridge.

Its meaning to you, however, is this: You can control the actions of your body. You can build in suggestions that will absolutely change your eating and drinking habits and cause you to lose weight.

The better you are able to raise your arm, the better you will be able to control your eating and drinking . . .

You may raise either your right arm or your left arm, whichever you choose, in the following fashion . . .

Raise either your right arm or your left arm about three inches at a time in a cogwheel-like fashion . . .

As your arm moves higher and higher with each cogwheel-like motion, your arm will get lighter and lighter—another sensation you are controlling . . .

Your arm is literally getting so light at this stage that you feel it may pull you up to the ceiling, like a balloon!

As your arm goes higher and higher the more deeply relaxed you will be . . .

You will raise your arm at the count of three . . . not because you have to, but because you really want to . . .

One . . . Two . . . Three . . .

Slowly the arm is lifting . . . lifting . . . lifting . . . and as it lifts higher . . . and higher . . . with each movement, your arm is getting lighter . . . and lighter . . . and lighter . . .

And as it gets lighter . . . and lighter . . . and lighter . . . notice how your state of relaxation is getting deeper . . . and deeper . . . and deeper . . .

No anxiety . . . feeling wonderful . . .

Your state of relaxation is getting deeper . . . and deeper . . . and deeper . . .

Just as your arm feels that it may float away, you will give youreelf another suggestion and surprise yourself again at the amount of control you have over your own body! From feeling an almost helium-like lightness, your arm will turn into a rigid extension that you can hold in a state of tension that is tighter and more durable than anything you can achieve while in a conscious state.

As your arm is getting into a perpendicular position, straight up, you will notice that you can develop another sensation . . . that of stiffness . . .

Your arm is now lifting higher and higher, so that your arm . . . fingers . . . hand . . . wrist . . . and forearm are stretched toward the ceiling . . .

Paradoxically, you will notice that the stiffer your arm gets from the fingers to the hand to the wrist to the elbow to the shoulder, the more deeply relaxed you will be . . .

Your arm is very stiff . . . very rigid . . . like a bar of steel . . . from the fingertips to the elbow to the shoulder . . .

Notice the stiffness of your outstretched arm . . .

You are doing fine . . .

By this point it will be clear to you when you're in the trance-state just how much power you really have over yourself and how easy it'll be to give yourself suggestions that will change your eating and drinking habits in a positive way. Compared to the dramatic physical state you have just caused your body to achieve, alteration of your other responses will be easy!

Now, if you wish to control still more symptoms, gain more mastery over your weight, and control your eating and drinking, at the count of three, about an inch or so at a time, allow your arm to fall to your side . . . and as your arm slowly falls, your arm will become limper and limper as it falls to your side . . .

Isn't it surprising how many feelings and sensations you are controlling and gaining control over? . . .

Isn't it remarkable how many sensations are built into your body and how you can control them? . . .

It sure is! You'll wonder why you didn't make these simple adjustments before!

Now, don't let your arm drop too rapidly . . . let it drop very . . . very . . . slowly . . .

In every movement of your arm going downward, suggest to yourself that when your arm reaches your side, it will be a signal for every muscle and every fiber in your body to develop a complete sense of relaxation . . .

One . . . two . . . three . . .

Now your arm is descending . . .

Slowly . . . slowly . . . slowly . . .

When it reaches your side, it will be a signal for every muscle in your body to relax completely . . .

Now you are in a very . . . very . . . deep state of relaxation . . . feeling no anxieties . . . feeling wonderful . . .

Now you have completed the induction of yourself into a trance-state when you will be feeling very relaxed and receptive to suggestions that you will make to yourself about the ways in which you will change your eating and drinking behavior. Your attention has closely focused on your own voice at this point, and as you listen to yourself make suggestions for future behavior (but during your "post-hyp" script), you will be struck by the simplicity and common sense of the things you are suggesting.

You know perfectly well the right way to eat and drink, and the reasons why you are not doing so. These are very obvious to you, and you will realize that the only person you are punishing with this behavior is yourself.

CHAPTER FOUR

STAIRWAY TO PARADISE

Relaxing deeply and focusing—in other words, self-hypnosis—can be achieved in a variety of ways. This induction script is simply another technique for you to use to put yourself in a deeply relaxed and receptive state of mind.

You may wish to try each of the induction scripts to find which works best for you, during the first few weeks.

This technique should be used while lying on a bed or sofa with your shoes off and any tight clothing loosened. Now, let's take a relaxing walk down the stairway!

As in all of these scripts, you should read the induction column in a low, soft monotone to yourself.

You're lying down with your eyes open, deeply relaxed . . .

And you begin to descend the stairway by taking a full, deep breath, and holding this breath in . . .

Filling your lungs to capacity . . .

You can still get a little more into your lungs . . .

You're feeling how tense holding your breath is making you . . .

Now you are realizing that when you let your breath out . . .

Every tension will be flowing out of you . . .

Like letting the air out of a balloon . . .

It's important to hold your breath for a considerable time feeling the tension in your body build and all your muscles tighten up from lack of oxygen.

You're letting your breath out now . . .

Feel it whoosh out . . .

Sinking as you do, very deeply, into a deep state of relaxation . . .

All tensions leaving your body . . .

Feeling very loose, very limp, very relaxed . . .

This breath-holding method of inducing relaxation quickly can be used during the day as a quick way to deal with anxieties and tension, to put yourself back into a calm mental state, and to remember the instructions you have given yourself while being relaxed. Now you go on to deepen your state of relaxation and to begin walking down the stairway.

You see yourself starting to walk down a long, dark stairway . . .

Very dark, so you can barely see anything ahead of you . . .

But this is comforting . . .

You are not afraid, knowing that you will soon be passing through the darkness . . .

Through the darkness of the negative attitudes that are causing your poor eating and drinking habits . . .

You are holding on to a stair railing and noticing how smooth it feels to your fingertips . . .

Hearing the sound of your footsteps on the carpeted stairs going down into the darkness . . .

With each step you are becoming even more deeply relaxed . . .

More deeply . . .

More deeply with each step on the stairs . . .

More deeply . . .

Now you are noticing that it seems to be getting lighter the deeper you go . . .

The light is sunlight . . .

Going deeper, and deeper, toward the sunlight . . .

Getting closer to the bottom . . .

Reaching the bottom, deeply relaxed . . .

One of the important elements of this induction is for you to recall vividly from your mind various tastes and smells. All of this information and the informa-

tion on how to eat correctly is already contained in that wonderful organ called the brain!

You see yourself stepping out into a lovely garden huge in scope . . .

The air is warm and summery . . .

You see the sunshine pouring down like honey . . .

And the smell of flowers is everywhere . . .

Orange trees ring the garden . . .

Deep green leaves with vivid oranges . . .

The smell of orange blossoms is heavy . . .

You smell the orange blossoms . . .

You hear the singing of a variety of birds and you can see the birds flying from tree to tree . . .

Hear the hummingbird nearby . . .

Colors of the flowers and the smell of the oranges . . .

Giving you much pleasure . . .

Relaxing you more deeply, even more deeply, even more deeply . . .

Now you see a beautiful little pond with lily pads and goldfish swimming underneath . . .

You feel wonderful . . .

So relaxed . . .

So at peace . . .

As all the sounds of the birds and the warmth of the sun make you feel so alive . . .

So free . . .

Now you're seeing a large shade tree with thick, deep green grass . . .

And you go to it . . .

A place to lie down . . .

Now you are lying down, looking up at the clear soft blue skies . . .

Now closing your eyes . . .

Feeling so much at peace . . .

So relaxed and at peace with the world . . .

Feeling so good . . .

So happy to be alive . . .

Finding yourself so full of life and vitality from now on . . .

Because now you are going to be more free from conflict . . .

From worry . . .

From frustration . . .

You are giving yourself some generalized instructions here that are important to you in changing your eating and drinking habits.

Many of these habits spring into place as a response to worry and anxiety.

Now you are going to be reacting positively and calmly to situations . . .

No longer pulled one way by your needs and another by your negative attitudes and fears . . .

No longer wasting energy, worrying or bottling things up inside you . . .

You're going to be feeling full of energy and life . . .

Liking yourself more . . .

Feeling relaxed and secure and confident . . .

Making others feel happy as well . . .

And making yourself all the happier as you create positive feelings in the people around you . . .

Feeling deeply relaxed . . .

No anxieties . . .

Feeling deeply at peace with yourself . . .

With one final breath-holding, you will be ready to begin your post-hypnotic suggestions to yourself.

You're taking in a full breath . . .

Holding it . . .

Holding it . . .

Filling your lungs to their complete capacity . . .

Squeezing in a little more air . . .

Holding it . . .

Noticing how tense you have become . . .

Feeling your muscles tighten . . .

Realizing how when you let your breath out . . .

All your tensions will be completely gone . . .

Letting your breath out . . .

Now! . . .

And sinking, sinking very deeply, very deeply to your deepest state of relaxation . . .

All your tensions are gone . . .

Extremely loose . . .

Very limp . . .

Ready to hear the ways you will eat and drink now in your new, exciting life.

You have at this point put yourself into a deeply relaxed and focused state and are ready to begin your post-hypnotic script which will tell you how to change your eating and drinking habits, resulting in losing weight, gaining great amounts of personal energy and vivacity, and leading a positive, new life!

CHAPTER FIVE

BREATHING AND COUNTING

In the following two chapters you will be able to learn short-cut techniques to relax during stressful times in your day—going in to ask the boss for a raise, giving an important party, speaking before a local club, and so forth.

Please note that the techniques in this chapter—quick, deep, breathing—should not be used by anyone who has had a history of epilepsy.

You will find that this particular means of relaxation is quick and effective, as the physical effects of hyper-oxygenating your system produces a relaxed state in short order, "kicking in" the state you have produced more slowly during your daily fifteen-minute session with your tape.

When you reach this relaxed state you will find that you also are "kicking in" the suggestions and advice you have given yourself in the post-hyp script, so that your positive new attitude and good eating and drinking behaviors are activated when you relax.

In this technique you take in fifteen full deep breaths in succession, very quickly, blowing out all the air after each breath and holding the last breath.

(Inhale) . . . One . . . (Exhale)

(Inhale) . . . Two . . . (Exhale)

(Inhale) . . . Three . . . (Exhale)

(Inhale) . . . Four . . . (Exhale)

(Inhale) . . . Five . . . (Exhale)

(Inhale) . . . Six . . . (Exhale)

(Inhale) . . . Seven . . . (Exhale)

(Inhale) . . . Eight . . . (Exhale)

(Inhale) . . . Nine . . . (Exhale)

(Inhale) . . . Ten . . . (Exhale)

(Inhale) . . . Eleven . . . (Exhale)

(Inhale) . . . Twelve . . . (Exhale)

(Inhale) . . . Thirteen . . . (Exhale)

(Inhale) . . . Fourteen . . . (Exhale)

(Inhale) . . . Fifteen . . .

(Hold your breath) . . .

You are feeling light-headed . . .

A tingling sensation . . .

Hearing your pulse beat . . .

Now you are letting out your final breath . . .

Sinking deeply . . .

Deeply . . .

To a wonderful state of relaxation . . .

Your body is completely loose . . .

Feeling wonderful . . .

That marvelous tingling all over . . .

Your mind is completely relaxed . . .

You have a wonderful, clean feeling as you feel the tingling going away . . .

In a matter of one minute, you can use this technique to rapidly relax yourself and "reinstate" the responses and positive attitudes you have been giving yourself in the fifteen-minute daily tape.

You are deeply relaxed now . . .

Realizing you have great control over your mind and your body . . .

Remembering how you will eat and drink . . .

Remembering your post-hyp instructions . . .

Happy and joyous in your new life . . .

This technique and the one in the next chapter *do not replace* your fifteen-minute daily tape. They are intended to augment your daily tape session to help you during stressful times during the day.

However, in a number of months, when you have successfully restructured your eating and drinking habits, you may find that a daily fifteen-minute tape session is no longer necessary, and these shorter relaxation methods may be used instead.

Taping it off not only works—it's fun! Like a mini-vacation!

CHAPTER SIX

PROGRESSIVE RELAXATION

In this method you tell yourself to progressively relax by focusing on different muscle groups in your body.

You will find this technique, once learned, is also excellent for producing a quick state of relaxation during the day by using a shortened version of the exercise. But first, let's relax!

As with the other scripts, you are reading this onto your tape in a low, soft voice, and in a monotone. You are lying on a bed, flat on your back, with a soft pillow under your head. As in other cases, you have removed your glasses or any contact lenses that you may be wearing.

You are lying on the bed, thinking of a pleasant, peaceful scene . . .

See yourself lying on the beach . . .

Feeling the warm sun on your face . . .

On your back, there is the gentle pressure of the soft, warm sand . . .

And you can see the blue cloudless sky . . .

And feel the warmth of the summer sun on your legs . . .

Now you are letting all the muscles of your body become limp and slack . . .

First, the muscles of your toes . . .

And your feet . . .

And your ankles . . .

Now you are letting them relax . . .

Letting them go . . .

Limp and loose and slack . . .

Next the muscles of your calves . . .

Letting them go . . .

Limp, loose . . .

Letting them relax . . .

Now the muscles of your thighs . . .

Letting them relax . . .

Feeling them let go . . .

Feeling them limp and slack . . .

As you can see, this technique produces the same deeply relaxed state as do the previous ones, but achieving this by focusing on muscle groups one at a time.

Now you are feeling a heaviness in your legs . . .

Your legs are feeling as heavy as steel girders . . .

Let your legs go even more . . .

Heavy as concrete piers . . .

Let them relax . . .

Completely relax . . .

As you relax your legs you are becoming sleepier and sleepier . . .

You feel no anxiety . . .

Completely at peace . . .

Your mind feeling calm . . .

Feeling contented . . .

You are greatly enjoying this very pleasant, relaxed, dowsy state of mind . . .

Now that the feeling of relaxation is spreading upward . . .

Taking over your whole body . . .

You are letting your stomach muscles relax . . .

Letting them go . . .

Limp and loose . . .

Now the muscles of your chest . . .

Your upper body . . .

The muscles in your back . . .

All of these are going limp and slack . . .

You are allowing them to completely relax . . .

Then this feeling of heaviness in your body . . .

Your body feeling enormously heavy . . .

As though it will sink through your bed . . .

Wanting to sink deeper and deeper . . .

Deep into the warm, soft sand . . .

Letting your body go . . .

Heavy as the heaviest metal . . .

Heavy as lead . . .

Letting your body sink comfortably . . .

Heavily into the sand . . .

And as it does so, you are feeling drowsier and sleepier . . .

Your eyelids are becoming heavier and heavier . . .

And your eyes more and more tired and sleepy . . .

Presently your eyes must close . . .

You cannot keep them open . . .

Now you feel they are having to close . . .

Just letting them go and you are just letting them go . . .

They close . . .

Entirely on their own . . .

This deep feeling of relaxation you are giving to yourself is one of the most pleasant sensations you'll experience . . .

To feel this deep relaxation every day for fifteen minutes will change your life! Just this feeling alone, and the knowledge that you can produce it whenever you want to, will improve your eating and drinking habits. But you will be giving yourself even more good sound advice!

Adjust, you are letting yourself relax . . .

More and more completely . . .

Feeling the heat of the summer sun coming down on your legs and on your forehead, on your cheeks . . .

Feeling warm and comfortable . . .

Completely at peace . . .

With this pleasant relaxing feeling now spreading into your neck . . .

And your shoulders . . .

Your arms . . .

Now you are letting those neck muscles relax . . .

Letting them go . . .

Limp and loose . . .

Feeling those neck and shoulder muscles completely loosening up . . .

Letting them relax . . .

And now the muscles in your arms . . .

Letting them relax . . .

Feeling them go limp and slack . . .

And now feeling that feeling of enormous heaviness in your arms . . .

As if your arms have been turned into lead weights . . .

Just letting your arms go limp . . .

Heavy as can be . . .

Feeling yourself relax them completely . . .

And as you do this . . .

Your eyes are becoming more and more tired . . .

So completely tired that they are closed . . .

Letting them close . . .

On their own . . .

Your eyes are closing now . . .

Closing . . .

Closing tighter and tighter . . .

So that they cannot be opened . . .

Feeling completely relaxed, deeply relaxed . . .

Ready to give yourself eating and drinking instructions . . .

When you have learned this technique thoroughly, you will be able to produce the same effects on yourself by a short cut described later.

Your new life is going to be relaxed, fulfilling, and satisfying!

CHAPTER SEVEN

THE CANDY LADY AND THE PIE GUY

This post-hyp script deals with a common situation with fat people—a food or foods that they simply love and eat too much of. For the purposes of illustration here we have chosen some foods that are often in the "downfall" category of fat folks.

However, obviously you will have your own foods to put in here which you and only you know too well!

This post-hyp script should be added to the induction script when you are assembling your very own script in Chapter Eighteen. Once you have achieved the deeply relaxed and focused state necessary to accept and retain suggestions, you begin to give yourself the kinds of suggestions and associations that you will have in the future with problem foods.

You will recall that this is called the "sensitization" technique, and you will learn how effective it is.

> If you really want to lose weight, you must simply change some of the foods that you eat for ones that are just as tasty, just as sweet, just as satisfying . . .
>
> You are going to picture now some of your favorite foods . . . foods that are causing you to be fat, or causing you poor health . . . foods that are causing you to shorten your life . . . foods that are causing you to be unattractive to look at . . .
>
> *These foods need not be limited to a single item, but should not comprise an endless list either. Concentrate on some two or three foods that are your major problems now. You can add and change these foods at a later time when you have changed your weakness for the ones you will mention in this first script.*

Think of the fresh doughnut smell in the bakery when you go in to buy the old fashioned doughnuts with the sugar glazing on them . . .

Think of the fresh chocolate doughnuts with the little chocolate drips coming down the sides . . .

Think of the chocolate eclairs with the cream filling . . . the squishy yellow custard with the sweet taste, and the sugary confection that gets on your fingers . . .

"Little chocolate drips" and the "squishy yellow custard" are important details here, and you should be very specific and suggestive in describing the foods you love and what it is about them that you love.

Picture yourself licking your fingers and eating these heavy, sugary, sweet, chocolate and custard eclairs . . .

Now think of yourself eating these foods while standing next to a mushroom plant . . .

Smell the sickening odor of the decaying mushrooms . . .

It doesn't have to be a mushroom plant! Think of something that has nauseated you with its taste or smell or looks. Imagining a mushroom plant won't be very effective for people who haven't smelled mushroom manure! Pick something that you have personally experienced as disgusting.

You feel very sick and nauseous . . .

You feel like throwing up . . .

You feel you can't eat another bite of this nauseous food that is making you fat and your body rotten, like the decayed mushrooms that are being made into manure for gardens . . .

Next, picture another favorite food . . .

See the jar of peanut butter sitting in the refrigerator . . .

See yourself loading the peanut butter onto a piece of soft, white bread . . .

Pile the peanut butter on . . .

Load it up very thickly . . .

See yourself biting into this soft, gooey, mixture of bread and peanut butter, and taste a strong peanut taste . . .

Now see yourself in the stables at the riding academy . . .

The more imaginative you can be in pairing problem foods with nauseous scents, the better. What you are trying to do here is create strong negative associations with your problem foods, and you need to personalize what these negative associations are so they're meaningful to you.

You are cleaning out the stables . . .

Smell the strong odor of horse manure as you are seeing yourself eat that peanut butter and bread . . .

It sickens you to think of eating that peanut butter and bread, knowing what it does to you and your body . . .

Next, see yourself sitting down in the middle of a vast, lovely, garden . . .

If, like one of the early Krupp munitions family, you enjoy the smell of stables, then this is not the right association for you!

What are your favorite fragrances? Use them here. If it is not jasmine, use the loveliest scent you know.

The smell of jasmine is everywhere and the air is warm . . .

The garden is on the edge of a sandy beach, and you see yourself walking down to the beach, wearing your bathing suit . . .

You feel the sun warm on your back in this setting, which is like a deserted beach on the Caribbean Sea, or a hidden beach on one of the Hawaiian Islands . . . the sand is warm under your bare feet and you feel the surf wash over your toes . . . the water is warm, like a lukewarm bath for your body . . .

As you walk along the water's edge and turn the corner of the beach, you see a door in a cliff surrounded by jasmine and honeysuckle . . .

The door is smooth and cool to the touch . . .

You open the door and see a long staircase curving down to a secret pool . . .

The water in the pool is green and warm, like the water of the ocean . . .

You close the door and descend the stairs . . .

With every step downward you become more and more relaxed . . .

When you reach the foot of the stairs you are in a deep state of relaxation . . .

And you are! You are in a profound trance here, ready to accept positive suggestions. It is important to give yourself positive suggestions in the post-hyp script as well as negative associations. You need to tell yourself not only what not *to do, but what wonderful new things to do* instead. *You must carry here a specific picture of yourself as you once were, or would like to be. See specifically where you are thin.*

You are standing at the foot of the stairs next to the pool . . .

The concrete around the pool is cool and rough to your feet . . .

All around the pool are baskets of honeysuckle and jasmine . . .

The smell is overpowering and marvelous . . .

You feel wonderful as you put your foot into the pool and feel the warm water . . .

You are alone and you take off your swimming suit, and you walk into the pool slowly . . .

You feel the warm, fragrant water lapping up your calves . . . up your thighs . . . soon you are walking in the pool and you are floating in the pool feeling how light your body is in the water . . .

When you get out you notice there is a large mirror at one end of the pool and you see yourself in this mirror . . .

The water drips off of your arms, on the tips of your fingers, and you are very warm . . . feeling wonderful . . .

You look at your body in the mirror carefully, one part at a time . . .

It is a very beautiful body . . . you feel very proud that you have it . . .

You are determined to take care of it . . .

On a table next to the mirror is your dinner . . .

On the plate on this table are chicken and fish and fresh vegetables . . .

On your plate we have put chicken and fish and fresh vegetables. You should be more specific than this, and put on your plate the kinds of foods that you will be eating in the near future. An idea of what these foods are is contained in the Appendix under the title "Some Good Foods and Recipes." You should talk here a little bit about how you will fix the chicken and with what kind of relishes, and how you will prepare the vegetables with a low-calorie sauce.

As you sit down to eat them, you can smell how good they are . . .

You see yourself eating these healthful foods . . . very slowly putting down your fork and spoon between each bite and chewing them very slowly . . .

This is very important. *People who eat their food slowly and put down their utensils between bites have been shown in many studies to be people in control of their weight. Rapid eating, or eating while standing, is the widespread behavior of fat people.*

You leave some of these vegetables and some of the fish and some of the chicken on your plate . . .

It is all right not to clean your plate . . .

Don't clean your plate! You don't have to eat all of your food. You are the boss, not the food!

For dessert another plate has fruits . . .

You have never tasted anything as sweet and fresh as this fruit . . .

It tastes marvelous. . . . and just a little of it gives you this feeling . . .

As you think of this dinner and the foods that you are eating, you also think of the best time that you can remember having had . . .

Think of it now . . .

You need to finish your post-hyp script with a positive association of yourself having an excellent time—getting some exciting news, having a peak emotional experience—and pairing this with the eating of healthful foods. For purposes of shorthand in this script, you are picturing yourself in a group of people having a marvelous time, but the important thing is for you to tell yourself and remind yourself when this happy time was. Obviously, it needn't have been in a group of people!

Picture it very specifically . . .

See the people laughing . . .

See the dresses and the suits they wore . . .

Feel the exhilaration you felt . . .

These times will come again . . . now that you're eating properly . . .

Those excellent times will soon be here . . .

At the end of every post-hyp script you must remember to bring yourself up out of the deeply relaxed state and to give yourself the instruction of energy and refreshment that you will feel when you wake up. Though no harm will befall you if you are interrupted in the middle of the trance session, this occurrence creates an "unresolved" feeling, with a certain amount of tension.

Now, at the count of three you are going to wake up feeling very refreshed . . . deeply relaxed . . . feeling wonderful . . . full of energy . . . full of positive feelings for the evening ahead . . .

One . . . two . . . three . . .

Eyes open . . . feeling wonderful . . . feeling relaxed . . .

When you combine your post-hyp script with the induction script in Chapter 3, allow yourself about forty-five minutes to dictate your own personal weight-loss cassette. Play this faithfully every evening, and you will lose weight without drugs, hunger pangs, or a feeling of deprivation. You will lose weight, and you will keep it off.

Perhaps even more importantly, you will learn a new series of responses to life's crises, and that may be the best news of all!

CHAPTER EIGHT

KITCHEN SNITCHIN'

Women, more often than not, have the additional temptation that comes with preparing meals and surviving in a kitchen environment.

Not only do meals have to be planned and fixed, they must be tasted! Worst of all, you must stay in the middle of this room with every possible eating temptation within four feet of your fingers at a time of day when you are yourself tired and hungry.

You can't pair up noxious smells and tastes with all the possible foods in your kitchen, because there are too many of them involved in the day-to-day preparation of meals, and you wouldn't want to feel that your entire kitchen smells bad in any event.

So for this particular, very common eating problem situation, you will use "positive imaging" techniques. You'll see yourself behave in a certain way in a very certain environment—your own kitchen. Your own kitchen, the most heavily used room in the house!

Positive imaging works extremely well in this situation because your familiarity with your own kitchen and the very "particular" characteristics of your kitchen give you the correct "cues" for your new behavior.

Along with seeing yourself behaving with pots and pans—and spoons!—in a positive way is the recall of times in your life when you felt marvelous. When you are in a deeply relaxed state, and you associate memories of very powerful "good times" with the correct kind of eating behavior, you'll find that this will ensure that kind of good behavior in the future.

And now, after you have read the induction script onto your tape to put you into a deeply relaxed and receptive state, read the script in the right-hand column as your post-hyp script and change for good! The post-hyp script in the right-hand column should be read into your tape immediately following your induction script.

Now you are remembering a time in your life when you felt the exhilaration of pure accomplishment . . .

You can see it as clearly now as when it happened to you . . .

You can remember the thrill it brought you . . .

The surge of blood within you . . .

The goose pimples . . .

Enormous feeling of expansion . . .

Achievement . . .

This experience in your life is not to be a long expansive time, but a specific event. Perhaps it was the time you were chosen as student body president, or the time you were praised for your work in front of the whole office; perhaps it is a memorable sexual experience. Whatever the experience you choose, it should be one in which the whole experience is exhilarating and in which there were no secondary negative feelings upon reflection. This experience or event should be a brief period of time. *Spend some time thinking about what your experience might be, your strongest "peak experience," and write this out in some detail before you dictate it onto your tape.*

And write it out in the present tense, *as though you are reliving the experience again right now.*

(Now write out this peak experience in the present tense and dictate it into your post-hyp script.)

You are seeing yourself in your kitchen . . .

Seeing it in very particular ways . . .

In the next paragraph of your script, fill in very specific details of your kitchen—the color of the paint and wallpaper, the texture of the counter top, the odor of the spice rack. You might wish to stand in your kitchen and list some of these specific physical descriptions. List six or eight of them. List how they look, taste; how they look, smell, sound.

(In this paragraph read in specific descriptions of your kitchen.)

And now you see yourself standing in your kitchen . . .

Feeling comfortable in your kitchen . . .

And relaxed . . .

You see yourself reflected in the kitchen window . . .

Seeing an image of yourself . . .

And you look thin . . .

You are looking very trim . . .

And enjoying the feeling immensely . . .

You look very fit and you are feeling fine . . .

Now you are seeing yourself making pies for a Thanksgiving dinner . . .

Feeling the pastry in your fingers . . .

As you put it in the pie plate . . .

Seeing the filling of lemon . . .

Of pumpkin . . .

And smelling how good their odors are . . .

Once again, you should imagine the kinds of desserts that you are fond of. You want to see yourself making a food that is tempting, and if you do not like lemon or pumpkin pies, that should be altered to apple or cherry or whatever flavor is your master!

You are seeing yourself making this pie . . .

But feeling no desire to taste it . . .

And its sight . . .

The smell of it . . .

And the feel of it in your hands makes you feel pleasant because someone else will enjoy eating it . . .

You will be giving pleasure to someone else whom you love . . .

But you see yourself . . .

Slim in the reflection from the kitchen window . . .

Finishing up making the pie . . .

And washing out the bowls . . .

Not licking them . . .

And putting the pie in the oven . . .

Feeling relaxed . . .

Feeling good about your slim self . . .

Now, in the next part of your post-hyp tape, describe yourself avoiding the foods you commonly eat while you are preparing dinner—mashed potatoes, perhaps wine while cooking, rolls or French bread in the oven, and other starches and sweets that you know quite well contain calories and put on pounds.

(Describe yourself avoiding these foods in the kitchen, and list the problem foods specifically.)

Now you are seeing yourself in your cozy kitchen . . .

Munching radishes and carrots . . .

And celery sticks . . .

And they are tasting marvelous . . .

Their flavors sharp and clean and rich . . .

You are salivating now . . .

Feel yourself salivating as you think of the highly desirable flavors of these radishes, carrots, and celery sticks . . .

Again, include other fresh vegetables that you like here, such as cucumbers, squash, and other green vegetables listed in the Appendix to this book.

You are seeing yourself in control of your kitchen . . .

And it is a marvelous feeling of accomplishment . . .

After dinner, you are seeing yourself scraping the plates and saving some food for casseroles or for family animals . . .

But you are not finishing uneaten food from the plates because it is "too good to waste" . . .

You feel that it is okay to leave food on the plates if you are not hungry . . . or give it to domestic pets . . .

And you are learning to prepare meals with smaller portions . . .

So there is less wasted food . . .

And you are feeling very smart . . .

And very positive about yourself . . .

Now . . .

Once more . . .

You remember that wonderful time in your life of exhilaration and accomplishments . . .

Feel it now . . .

Surging through you . . .

And remember that you can do whatever you set out to do in controlling your food and eating habits . . .

Now you will give yourself a few reminder suggestions before awakening yourself.

Since you really wish to lose weight, you will roll the food in your mouth at dinner from the front of the tongue to the back of the tongue and from side to side . . .

To obtain the most satisfaction from each bite you eat . . .

Satisfying the thousands of taste buds located on your tongue . . .

Finding that less food is required . . .

And calories eaten dramatically reduced . . .

Next you will keep an image of yourself in your mind . . .

Of how you once looked when you were thin . . .

If you have a good picture of yourself when you were thin, place it on your bulletin board or on the front of the refrigerator so that you can be reminded of how you looked, and how you will look again!

Next, think of the worst, most nauseous smell that you have ever experienced . . .

Perhaps rotten eggs . . .

Perhaps seasickness, perhaps the results of a time when you were seasick . . .

And in the future, when you desire to eat something fattening and not good for you . . .

You will instantly associate this disagreeable odor with that food . . .

And also, the revolting taste of soured milk . . .

Can be associated with these fattening foods when you simply think of them . . .

Buy the most beautiful dress you can afford . . .

At least two sizes too small for you . . .

And hang it in your bedroom where you can see it every morning . . .

And see yourself getting into this dress in a short time . . .

In the case of men, substitute the thought of a favorite old sports jacket now too small, or a tuxedo, or tennis shorts that no longer fit. But most important of all, see yourself wearing those clothes in a short time, and think how happy you will be!

Now, at the count of three you are going to wake up feeling very refreshed . . .

Deeply relaxed . . .

Feeling wonderful . . .

Full of energy . . .

Full of positive feelings for the evening ahead . . .

One . . .

Two . . .

Three . . .

Eyes open . . .

Feeling wonderful . . .

Feeling realxed .

If you combine this script with the induction script in Chapters 3 through 6, you will have produced a powerful learning tape that will reshape your eating habits. Play this faithfully every evening. You will lose weight, without any feeling of being deprived. You will, in fact, *TAPE IT OFF!*

CHAPTER NINE

AT THE TABLE

You need not only to control *what* you eat, however. As important, and perhaps more important, are *where* and *how* you eat.

Sitting in the kitchen while you are fixing dinner, watching television, or reading the newspaper at a luncheonette or fast food place—all of these are the wrong sort of "how." Eating should be an event in itself, not something done while you are drowsing along in a half-fantasy state of mind, gathering wool or counting your worry beads.

You should eat sitting down at a table that is used regularly for that purpose, if possible, not at a variety of places. However, in today's work-a-day world, this is not always possible, and the next best situation is to remember not to eat on the run. Eating fast or too quickly is a sure-fire way to take on more calories, because your taste buds don't have a chance to savor the food and gain the full satisfaction from it.

It is important to understand that eating is suggested to you by many things other than hunger pangs in the stomach, and if you are in the habit of having a piece of pie in front of the fire or eating on television trays in front of the set, these surroundings will act as signals to you in the following way: Picture yourself in front of the fire about 9 PM, feeling tired from the day's activities, and perhaps a little bored, perhaps even a little worried about your child's grades in high school, and the rumor that some new illicit substance is now being smoked behind the gymnasium. The fire is warm and cozy and you think to yourself, "Wouldn't it be nice to have a piece of pie here in front of the fire?"

You don't feel any hunger pangs in your stomach, but you are responding to a signal from your environment to combine multiple pleasures (eating, coziness, warmth) to overwhelm your anxiety and fatigue.

Eat only at the table!

You should eat only at regular times, as well, because hunger pangs themselves are not the work of some little leprechaun in your stomach who demands food. You feel hunger according to what times you are accustomed to eating, and if you snack throughout the day at unpredictable times, you will condition yourself to feel small, but nearly continuous, signals to eat.

Three good meals a day remain important, as you always learned they were. Breakfast is especially important, and is the most-abused mealtime. *Don't skip breakfast!* The food you eat at breakfast—and to a lesser extent, lunch—is utilized that day by your body.

In short, these are the mechanics of eating:

WHO	*You*
WHAT	The right stuff (and you know what it is, but the Appendix reminds you)
WHERE	Seated at the table or counter where you regularly eat
WHEN	Three times a day with a good breakfast, a good lunch, and a light dinner
HOW	Slowly chewing each bite at least twenty times, and doing nothing except conversing with eating companions (no reading, or television watching)
WHY	Because you feel hunger pangs, and *not* because of feelings of anxiety, depression, anger, frustration, or boredom.

In the following script, you will learn a technique, and give yourself suggestions, to stop inappropriate "hunger pangs" you may be feeling because of conditioning you have given yourself to eat throughout the day. This hypnotic technique is called "glove anesthesia." In addition, you will see yourself in this script eating in the correct way, and experience the power of taping it off!

In a low monotone, read the following script onto your tape following the induction script. Although "glove anesthesia" refers to the numbing effect that can be produced on a hand, you'll see that you can produce a similar effect in your stomach.

You are very relaxed in a cabin high in the Swiss Alps . . .

It is very dark, near midnight . . .

You hear the wind howling, and moaning outside the window . . .

But you are sitting beside a fireplace inside . . .

Staring deeply into the coals . . .

Feeling the heat from the fire radiating out . . .

Feeling the warmth and the flames against your skin . . .

Feeling the prickling, almost itching feeling in your thighs from the heat from the fire . . .

You are seeing the flickering shadows from the fire on the wall . . .

Hearing the popping and snapping of the logs as they burn . . .

You smell the smoke from the burning fire . . .

And the room is dark except for the light from the fire . . .

It is very quiet . . .

You rise from the chair . . .

You are going outside . . .

Out into the cold night . . .

And you dress up with a sweater . . .

And a heavy coat . . .

You put on gloves, a cap, and heavy boots . . .

And go to the door.

You feel the door yield to the pressure of your hand.

You are outside in the cold winter air.

You take a deep breath of cool fresh mountain air.

You smell the pine forests.

You feel so good breathing in this pure fragrant air.

Your whole rib cage collapses in total relaxation.

You hear the door as you close it.

The moon is full and silver.

Outside it is ten degrees below zero, terribly cold.

You see your breath as it comes out of your mouth.

You begin walking down a path, and on either side you see tall, deep pine trees covered with snow.

The snow is almost hip deep, and everything has a blue-black shade to it, even the snow.

Ten minutes pass.

Twenty minutes pass.

Thirty minutes pass.

You stop, and take the glove off your right hand and thrust your warm hand into the snow . . .

Making a fist . . .

Compressing the snow into a snowball . . .

Terribly cold . . .

In the palm of your hand . . .

You feel a numb . . .

Wooden . . .

Leather-like sensation beginning in your right palm . . .

Spreading throughout your hand.

When you feel this sensation, you place your right hand upon your stomach.

Now you let all that numb feeling drain from your hand into your stomach . . .

Your stomach is becoming numb, leathery, wooden . . .

Just as if Novocain had been injected into it . . .

Feeling like your jaw at the dentist after the tingling has worn off . . .

Numb and wooden . . .

Your hand is now becoming warm and alive again and you can feel the blood rushing into it.

When all the numbness has drained from your hand into your stomach, place your right hand again at your side.

After a moment place your right hand on your stomach once again, and let all the numb feelings in your stomach drain back into your hand.

You hand is becoming numb, leathery, like a piece of wood, and your stomach is becoming warm, flushed, with feelings once again, as the blood rushed back through the veins surrounding it. When all that numbness has drained from your stomach back to your hand, put your hand again at your side.

You are doing fine!

Now you put your glove back on your right hand again.

Put it on.

You turn around and begin tracing your footsteps back to your mountain cabin.

Ten minutes pass.

Twenty minutes pass.

Thirty minutes.

You are back to the cabin, you go inside, where you take off all your outer boots and gloves and walk over to the fire.

Hold your hands over the fire, feel its warmth spreading throughout your body.

All your body feels warm and cozy.

The warmth of the fire and the smell of its smoke, the snapping and the popping of the logs, and the moaning of the wind.

All these sensations seem far, far away as you drift deeper and deeper, feeling very relaxed, feeling wonderful.

You've now shown yourself the control you have over sensations in your body! Now you will give yourself some correct eating instructions with the use of a new friend—glove anesthesia.

Now see yourself sitting down, at a table, eating your breakfast . . .

Your lunch . . .

Your dinner.

You are feeling relaxed and calm.

As you sit down, you quickly tighten all your muscles, taking a deep breath . . .

Hold this tension for a count of three . . .

And releasing the tension and letting out your breath quickly . . .

You are feeling deeply relaxed and happy . . .

For the first five or six weeks, it is very helpful to keep a "food diary" of all the food you eat, both the kind and the quantity. This should be written down before you begin eating. *A food diary will not only give you a clear picture of what sort of fuel you are putting into your body, it will also act in what psychologists call a "secondary reinforcing manner," and you will find yourself eating less and screening out fattening foods by virtue of writing them down on this paper. Even though no one but yourself is going to read this diary, you will find yourself mildly disgusted at having to write down a problem food.*

See yourself taking a bite of food . . .

Putting your fork down on your plate . . .

And taking your hand away from your fork . . .

Chewing the food thoroughly . . .

Tasting it, by rolling the food from the front of the tongue to the back of the tongue and from side to side and tasting the last ounce of satisfaction and the last drop of flavor out of each morsel.

By chewing slowly and rolling the food around over the thousands of taste cells on your tongue, less food will be required and you will more easily satisfy (that is to say, overload) these taste cells. You'll find that less food is required, and your calorie intake dramatically reduced. For most people, this technique itself is the most important in losing weight, rather than eliminating problem foods.

But when you restrict the place and manner of your eating to the dinner table, and *eliminate "emotional eating,"* and *change or reduce problem foods—your "weight problem" is over!*

Now you are reacting in a positive way to some remarks that your meal companion has made . . .

Not discussing problems while you eat . . .

Not talking of difficulties which create tensions while you eat . . .

And chewing and swallowing your food before you speak . . .

Not only because it is polite to do so . . .

But because it slows down the ingestion of food . . .

And gives your body a chance to be satisfied . . .

Now see yourself at the weight you need to be . . .

Trim and looking good . . .

Admired by others . . .

Relaxing and feeling wonderful . . .

Knowing that the weight you need to lose will come off . . .

At a healthful rate . . .

And see yourself . . .

Somewhat surprised that you cannot eat everything on your plate . . .

That you are not that hungry . . .

And knowing that it is all right to leave food on your plate . . .

It is okay . . .

And you will be learning not to waste food as you give yourself smaller portions . . .

Because you are not as hungry . . .

And knowing that it's all right to stop eating when you are full . . .

For those times when you think you are hungry because you feel "hunger pangs"—particularly late in the evening for many people—give yourself the instruction in the right-hand column.

Between meals, and in the evening after dinner . . .

If you feel something that resembles what you used to think was a hunger pang . . .

You will remember the numbness and wooden feeling of your hand . . .

Placing it on your stomach . . .

And feeling the numbness drain into your stomach . . .

So that your stomach now feels nothing . . .

It's completely numb . . .

Feeling like your jaw after Novocain has been injected and the tingling has gone away . . .

Completely numb.

Now, at the count of three you are going to wake up feeling very refreshed . . .

Deeply relaxed . . .

Feeling wonderful . . .

Full of energy . . .

Full of positive feelings for the evening ahead . . .

One . . .

Two . . .

Three . . .

Eyes open . . .

Feeling wonderful . . .

Feeling relaxed . . .

This chapter is one of them most important in the book for most people in changing their eating and drinking behavior, and you will find that it will change yours in a short space of time. You will find yourself behaving positively at the table, and eating in a different way. Habits are learned and can be changed, and you will change yours!

CHAPTER TEN

SEX IS SCARY

Like domestic conflict in a later chapter, sex can be the source of frustration, leading to the refrigerator, either:

- lack of sex, or
- quality of sex, or
- fear of sex.

Fat can even be a form of faithfulness, a defense against sexual advances by parties other than the fat person's spouse.

You may find overeating, and the accompanying fat produced, to be a subtle defense against becoming involved with a member of the opposite sex, since if you are fat—presumably—few people will desire you in a sexual sense, and the question of having sex will thus not arise.

Many people feel unloved and unlovable because of some characteristics about their own bodies that, in their eyes, seem to guarantee sexual rejection. So eating and drinking too much and putting on fat can be a clever way of assuring themselves that they will never face sexual humiliation about breasts, genitalia, or facial features. The fat, in a sense, acts as a shield or outer defense for greater fear. Fat, after all, is a common and widespread condition, an accepted way of putting yourself on the sexual shelf.

Certainly we all have factors in our early lives that affect the way we feel about sex; not all of these are positive. But you don't have to hang onto these early experiences for the rest of your life. You have in your hands a powerful means to change old attitudes and responses!

First of all, read an induction script into your tape, and then pick up the narrative of this script, remembering to read in a low monotone.

You find yourself standing in a huge garden . . .

In complete darkness . . .

With a summery, tropical feeling . . .

A hidden garden in Hawaii . . .

All alone . . .

With a full moon in the sky through the palm trees . . .

Deep in the interior . . .

With the air warm and balmy . . .

You are seeing the yellow moon . . .

And smelling the powerful fragrance of orange blossoms . . .

Picking an orange off the tree . . .

Feeling its pebbly skin . . .

You are now peeling off some of the orange rind, and biting deeply into the ripe orange . . .

Taste the tart sweetness . . .

Walking deeper and deeper into the garden . . .

Seeing lemon trees, yellow in the full moonlight . . .

And picking a lemon . . .

Smelling its tart fragrance by the stem . . .

Peeling a piece of its skin and smelling the lemony odor . . .

Now you bite deeply into the lemon . . .

Puckering your mouth as the sour lemon juice fills your mouth . . .

You see long descending alabaster stairs bright white in the full moon . . .

You are descending the stairs . . .

Feeling more deeply relaxed with every step . . .

More deeply relaxed . . .

When you reach the bottom of the stairs you are in a profound state of relaxation . . .

Now you are standing at the foot of the stairs . . .

A large marble swimming pool is in front of you, and around the pool are red and yellow roses in the moonlight . . .

And the smell of these roses clings in the air . . .

You are taking off your clothes . . .

You slide into the pool slowly . . .

Feeling the warm water come up your calves . . .

your thighs . . .

your hips . . .

To your waist . . .

And now you are floating on your back in the warm water smelling the heavy rose scent, looking up at the full moon . . .

Now you are walking up out of the pool . . .

Standing up you see a large mirror at one end of the pool and see your reflection in the glass . . .

Look at your body . . .

At this point you are to visualize your body at the proper weight you are going to reach soon. Perhaps the weight you once were, but in any case a realistic, healthful weight for you. (These "desirable weights" are contained in the Appendix.)

Look at the image in the mirror carefully . . .

See the trim waistline . . .

The firm thighs . . .

The clean chin line . . .

You are feeling very proud of your body . . .

You run your hands over it, feeling wonderful about yourself . . .

This is the body your new eating and drinking habits will give you . . .

And you feel marvelous . . .

As noted before, the number of sexual frustrations that may result in overeating and drinking are many and varied: Not enough sexual activity, incomplete sexual activity failing to result in orgasm, a feeling that sexual activity is unpleasant or distasteful, or a fear of rejection because of a feeling of inadequacy about one's body. These by no means exhaust the list but are among the most common. Sexual problems (such as impotence, premature ejaculation, frigidity, dyspareunia and vaginismus) are treatable by hypnobehavioral therapy on an individual basis, and if any of these is troubling you, you should seek professional help.

This post-hyp script deals with body image.

Gradually you are aware that you are not alone in the garden . . .

There are many others in the garden looking at you admiringly . . .

Smiling and nodding their heads . . .

Approving of your attractive body . . .

You are feeling marvelous!

Whenever you feel the impulse to eat or drink badly, you will remember this—the image of your beautiful body in the warm, summer eve in the garden.

Now, at the count of three you are going to wake up feeling refreshed . . .

Deeply relaxed . . . feeling wonderful . . .

Full of energy . . . and positive feelings about the evening ahead . . . and tomorrow . . .

One . . . two . . . three . . .

Eyes open!

Feeling wonderful . . .

Feeling relaxed and energetic.

Feelings of physical inadequacy and fear of the opposite sex—which after all are secondary to hunger—can be changed through consistently applying the techniques in *TAPE IT OFF!* You'll be more relaxed and accepting of yourself, and so will others!

CHAPTER ELEVEN

HASSLES AT WORK

Food and drink can be used as a tool to forget tough times at the office, as well.

In a symbolic way, it can be a means of armoring yourself against the slings and arrows of outrageous fortune hunters, and its saddest form shows itself in the case of the poor soul taking vodka with his or her orange juice in the morning before work.

The variety of displeasures you may feel at work are so numerous that we can't list them all, but certainly include feelings of being unappreciated, of being picked upon, of worrying about younger competition, loss of status within the office, and loss of your job. Ask yourself if problems at work are one of the causes for your poor eating and drinking behavior. Basic to any weight and fitness program is some honest self-analysis; for a period of two weeks, keep some informal notes on a few sheets of paper you assign to that purpose, reporting your eating and drinking behavior. When do you eat? What do you eat? What are your problem foods? Where do you eat? (The latter is very important.)

Most important of all: What's on your mind while you eat? If you were eating with someone else in a "private" manner—eating too quickly, eating the wrong foods, washing the food down with coffee or too much wine—what are you talking about with this person, and what is making you nervous? If you are eating alone, what are you dreaming about? (Problem eating, as we said before, is usually "soothing" a troubled emotional state; so what were you thinking or talking about before you started eating that peanut butter and jelly sandwich?)

Once you have identified some of your bad eating behaviors, you can use a tape to change them! Remember, you have no secrets from yourself. But the mind is ingenious in throwing up various camouflages for your behavior. So be honest with yourself; there's no one else around you have to fool or mislead.

If your problem turns out to be one generated by the work you are doing for a living, write it down, and you will use it later in this book. We do not deal here with the work-place situation itself, in the same way that we do not deal with the counseling that is likely to be necessary in domestic or marital problems. Professional counseling should be sought to take up problems involving groups of people, whether it's the marital group of two or the office group of five hundred.

What *TAPE IT OFF!* will do is improve your reactions to many of the seemingly "external" situations that we take up in this book, and make you a calmer, more positive person in your reactions to life's merry-go-round!

In a low monotone, read the following material onto your tape following one of the induction scripts given earlier. This text has the effect of deepening and intensifying the suggestions you will give yourself near the end of the script.

You are very, very relaxed . . .

Ten minutes on the clock will seem like one minute to you . . .

Times goes by very rapidly . . .

Seeming almost like an instant . . .

Too short to measure . . .

In less than one hour you can accomplish your entire day's work . . .

And accomplish it very effectively . . .

Understanding it and completing it more effectively than you normally would . . .

So relaxed and focused are you . . .

In addition to deepening your relaxation state, this part of the script will give you a time-shortening ability, so that your perception of difficult times can be shortened. This kind of approach has worked well with people who dread long ship voyages or flights in aircraft.

You are in a room on the second story of a large home . . .

In the still of the deep night . . .

And you're looking out a large window with heavy black velvet curtains . . .

You see the moonlight pouring in . . .

Lighting the room almost as brightly as day . . .

You see a bed much like the bed you slept in when you were ten years old . . .

And the boys of your tenth year are sitting on a table near the bed . . .

Outside is the street with a clock tower . . .

A winding stream shining silver in the moonlight . . .

A bridge . . .

And rolling countryside.

Now the clock is beginning to strike the hour of midnight . . .

It strikes for the first time. You see clouds drifting over the moon . . .

Making the clouds transparent . . .

The clock strikes a second time.

A warm wind blows in the window . . .

Pushing the heavy velvet curtains against your arm . . .

The wind brings the smell of crops ripening in the springtime . . .

On the third strike of the clock you smell the sweet heavy scent of star jasmine . . .

The clock strikes for the fourth time, and you hear a dog barking beneath your window . . .

On the fifth strike on the clock you notice the taste of honey from the tea and honey you had after dinner . . .

On the sixth strike of the clock you look outside and see a series of sparklers, like the sort you used as a child on the Fourth of July.

The clock strikes for the seventh time.

The sparkle from the sparklers comes into the room, filling it with a golden glow . . .

On the eighth strike of the clock you feel a sensation of weightlessness . . .

The idea of weightlessness is a very important one to people feeling the pressure of external events and people. Weightlessness is nothing more than the absence of external forces, and when you are able to call up this feeling quickly, it will be very useful to relax yourself!

Feel yourself with no weight at all . . .

When the clock strikes for the ninth time, you feel your body carried upward and floating out the window . . .

And the tenth sound of the clock seems very distant indeed . . .

So far away you can barely hear it . . .

On the eleventh chime you hear a far away dog bark, and the bark sounds little more than a yelp . . .

When the clock strikes the hour of midnight you remember all kinds of happy childhood memories . . .

Cotton candy at the fair . . .

Christmas days of your youth . . .

The happy thrill of the ferris wheel . . .

The excitement of Easter egg hunts . . .

You are floating over your city over the river and the countryside . . .

And then straight up toward the stars . . .

You are extremely relaxed.

The variety of pressures you can feel at work, as we've said, are many and varied. However, mostly they boil down to one or more unpleasant personalities with whom you must deal. Personnel conflict and boredom (either with repetitive work or with being too long in the same job) are the most common job complaints—except, of course, getting fired!

We are going to assume that the work place problem facing you in this particular script is that of a younger co-worker who is overextending himself and trying to become your supervisor.

You see the face of George Jones, a smart aleck youngster at the desk next to yours who treats you like his slave . . .

See the features on his face clearly . . .

See his irritating smile . . .

Hear the tone of his voice and the accent of his words as he throws some papers on your desk and tells you to finish them up . . .

Now see yourself watching him out the door, and feel the terrible urge for a doughnut . . .

And maybe not one doughtnut but two . . .

See yourself going to the coffee room and the doughnut box . . .

See yourself looking at the variety of doughnuts in the box . . .

The jelly doughnuts . . .

The chocolate doughnuts . . .

The old-fashioned glazed doughnuts . . .

And the cinnamon doughnuts . . .

You see yourself picking a custard doughnut out of the box . . .

Smelling it . . .

And then you see yourself putting the doughnut away . . .

Replacing it carefully . . .

Putting down the napkin . . .

And walking away . . .

You feel marvelous! . . .

Deeply relaxed with a feeling of exaltation . . .

And you see yourself in a mirror in the coffee room sideways as you leave . . .

And you notice how trim and thin you are . . .

And you know that you have won . . .

You are relaxed and positive to other people . . .

And you stop at another worker's desk . . .

And compliment her on the way she looks today . . .

You cheer her up . . .

Make her feel better . . .

And you feel much better yourself . . .

Maybe the temptation isn't doughnuts. Whatever the temptation or problem food is that you resort to after encounters with George, this is the food behavior to "extinguish." If there are two or three, go on to list these as well, always rewarding yourself with an excellent feeling and the pleasure of yourself as a fit person, after you have seen yourself taking avoidance behavior and not stuffing that forbidden food or drink into your mouth.

However, one of the most common reasons for a frustrated feeling at work is the inability of people to say what is on their minds in a positive, assertive way without being "offensive." Timidity is an accessory to frustration, and for that reason, to fatness. So try visualising yourself saying what you feel to George in a positive, yet firm way.

You see George Jones coming up to your desk, once again, about to hand you some work he should be doing . . .

Or to tell you to do your work in another way, correcting your behavior and overstepping his authority . . .

Listen to the irritating nasal twang in his voice . . .

See the insinuating smile on his lips . . .

The freckles on his nose . . .

And see him perching on the edge of your desk as he prepares to tell you how to do your job.

When he is through you see yourself saying to him the following statement: "George . . .

Thanks for your advice . . .

But I have my own job to do . . .

You are not my supervisor . . .

And I suggest you take care of your own work . . .

Just so we understand one another: I'm not your secretary. However, I'll be happy to cooperate on the Thingamajig Project and do my share."

Finish on a positive note, but give him clear boundaries, so that your relationship is clearer.

You see yourself looking him firmly in the eye . . .

Seeing his surprised expression . . .

And you feel a feeling of exaltation . . .

Joyous . . .

As you realize that George now knows he cannot push you around . . .

You are feeling marvelous . . .

And relaxed . . .

And in control . . .

And the last thing you want is something to eat . . .

You celebrate with your friend by going roller skating for lunch . . .

The more detail you can add about your work station, and the particular person causing frustration the better and more effective you will be at producing in yourself the right response to change your eating and drinking behavior.

Now, at the count of three you are going to wake up feeling very refreshed . . .

Deeply relaxed . . .

Feeling wonderful . . .

Full of energy . . .

Full of positive feelings for the evening ahead . . .

One . . .

Two . . .

Three . . .

Eyes open . . .

Feeling wonderful . . .

Feeling relaxed . . .

As mentioned before, problems in life—and certainly in the work place—are very common and produce feelings of frustration for many people. What you will now be able to do is to react positively to these feelings of frustration, with a greater feeling of confidence in yourself!

It is very important that you play these tapes on a daily basis during the first few weeks so that they can take affect, and in the case of a Hassle at Work it may help to play this to yourself before you go to work in the morning or during your lunch hour.

But you will now be able to focus your attention on work itself, and to speed the workday up through time-shortening concentration—and through *TAPE IT OFF!*

This *works.*

CHAPTER TWELVE

DOMESTIC DISSENT

Food and alcohol, as you well know, can be used as crutches or as a kind of consolation when some part of your life is not going the way you would like it to go.

This use of food to counter a feeling of frustration, in fact, is probably the most common problem in weight management. After all, food and drink are readily available, satisfying, can be consumed in almost any kind of social situation, and are available in a wide range of prices. You don't have to be wealthy to be fat!

Although this chapter will show you how to deal with one form of frustration—when married life is something of a strain—the techniques used in this post-hyp script can be used when frustration, for whatever reason, is the main cause of your bad eating and drinking behavior. In this script, you will focus on providing "replacement behaviors" in times of emotional trouble.

Put another way: When times get tense, you will get rid of that refrigerator reach and give yourself a new response! As with other post-hyp scripts, you will read this into your tape recorder immediately following an induction script. Read this in a low voice in a monotone.

You are feeling very relaxed . . .

Warm . . .

In a snug bed . . .

With a deep, soft comforter . . .

Listening to the early morning sounds in a little house in the country . . .

In the very early morning . . .

Feeling very snug . . .

And going back to sleep . . .

Perhaps this is your grandmother's house out in the country, or that of your aunt. Maybe it is a vacation cabin on a lake when you were young and your impressions of the world vivid.

You stretch . . .

Feeling luxurious and deeply relaxed . . .

Getting out of bed as the sun is rising . . .

The sky is turning the colors of the rainbow . . .

Going into the kitchen . . .

Following your nose . . .

The glorious smell of bacon . . .

And a plate of fried eggs . . .

With the bakery smell of hot homemade biscuits . . .

And a bowl of farm butter . . .

Feel your teeth sinking into the bacon . . .

Hearing it crunch . . .

Tasting its flavor . . .

And all the salty taste of the butter . . .

On the sourdough biscuits . . .

You will notice as you describe marvelous foods that your mouth will begin to salivate! This is simply one more proof that you are able to give your body suggestions on which it will act. You can "turn on" sensations of hunger, and you can turn them off, too.

Outside, the summer morning is warm . . .

Feel the warmth on your forearms . . .

With just a slight edge of early morning coldness . . .

Looking at the vivid colors of the morning . . .

The calico cat . . .

The vegetable garden with its reds . . .

Oranges . . .

Greens . . .

And the blue sky overhead . . .

Hearing the voices of children, laughing . . .

You sit on the comfortable old sofa next to the old ticking clock . .

Hearing the clock tick . . .

Listening to the passing of time . . .

Hearing the tick . . .

Tock . . .

Tick . . .

Tock . . .

Watching the deep blue sky . . .

Noticing that your stomach after a long time . .

Feels hungry . . .

You are getting up and going into the kitchen . . .

And picking up a biscuit still on the platter . . .

With butter melted into its crevices . . .

Taking a single bite . . .

Feeling your teeth sink through the biscuit and meet each other . . .

Tasting the marvelous biscuit-butter flavor . . .

And a suspicion of strawberry . . .

Taste the strawberry . . .

Then back outside to the comfortable old sofa . . .

And listening to the clock tick . . .

Tock . . .

Tick . . .

Tock . . .

Feeling the texture of the old rough wood arms on the sofa . . .

The soft weather-beaten cushions . . .

Hearing a dog barking in the distance . . .

Staring up at the blue sky . . .

Finding yourself drifting . . .

This "deepening image" is universal and general in nature. It can be strengthened in your own highly personal script, adding details of a specific relaxing place—whether it's your grandmother's house or a vacation cabin—that you have experienced in your own life. The details should be specific and pleasant and true to your own memory. They should include memories of all of your senses: sight, sound, touch, taste, and smell.

You go for a stroll in a field of thick, knee-high green grass . . .

Fragrant and fresh smelling . . .

Hearing the sounds of birds, of crows cawing in the distance . . .

Picking a blade of grass and tasting its freshness and vitality . . .

And then lying down in the grass . . .

Feeling its cushioning, pillowy effect . . .

Looking up at the blue sky . . .

On a lazy summer day . . .

Feeling yourself drifting and relaxed in every fiber of your muscles . . .

Half asleep . . .

With no worries . . .

At this point in your script you have relaxed yourself very deeply and you are ready to give yourself instructions for replacement behavior when you encounter frustrations.

In the script shown at the right, some common domestic disagreements are used to illustrate what your script should contain. However, it is important that you list domestic conflicts that you are experiencing. *List two or three of the conflicts that are most important, and which* immediately *precede your reach for the food crutch.*

It is important for you to think about this a bit, and not select some of the minor irritations contained in most marriages; for example, probably it is a greater conflict than socks on the bedroom floor or panties in the shower that is causing you to go for the refrigerator. Focus on major conflict areas.

See yourself with your partner, in a typical domestic quarrel . . .

Seeing the two of you in a familiar setting . . .

Noticing the furniture . . .

Hearing your partner's voice . . .

With that irritating tone of voice . . .

Telling you, of all people . . .

That you don't know how to manage money and never will . . .

When he just bought himself a new set of power tools . . .

Again, choose areas of domestic conflict that are true in your case. Money management, sexual selfishness, and child raising are the classic domestic battlegrounds—never forgetting relations with in-laws!

But choose your own area here, and be vivid in recalling the details of the conflict.

Listen to him lecturing you on balancing the checkbook . . .

Feel your anger rising from the injustice of this . . .

See the superior smile on his face . . .

Feel the impulse to throw something . . .

Which you barely control . . .

Listening to him lecture you on how hard it is to earn money . . .

When you're earning almost as much as he is . . .

And running the house as well . . .

As though he ever washed any dishes . . .

Suddenly you see yourself starting to talk and saying things you know will make him angry . . .

Asking him where the bonus was that he said would be coming in . . .

And what he intended to do with those power tools . . .

How you had been intending to save money for Christmas . . .

And how he spent it on himself instead . . .

Then seeing him grab his jacket and go out the front door . . .

Slamming it . . .

And knowing that he is going down to the village pub . . .

Where that busty barmaid works . . .

Again, these particular conditions may not match your domestic dissent at all. It would be miraculous if they matched it closely enough for you to use this without making some changes. But by this time in your script, you should be feeling some of the tension that you would be feeling in your own real life problem situation, if you have described it well.

This is the time, in real life, that you would be heading for the kitchen, still angry, not specifically thinking about getting something to eat, perhaps only with the idea of putting something away in the refrigerator or cleaning up the dishes as your mind, still outraged, reviews all the unfair and terrible conditions of life you are confronting.

But your feelings of anger will not permit you to go into the kitchen . . .

There is an invisible wall in the doorway leading to the kitchen . . .

And you cannot cross it . . .

It is as though a flashing sign . . .

In large red letters . . .

Said "Do not go into the kitchen" . . .

Because if you go into the kitchen . . .

He will win the argument . . .

And you don't want him to win the argument . . .

And you don't want him to have the last word . . .

And that is what he will be having if you go into the kitchen . . .

Instead . . .

You find yourself going into the bedroom . . .

And taking the rug you have been braiding out from under the bed . . .

And sitting down . . .

Turning on a radio station you enjoy . . .

And braiding that rug furiously . . .

Pulling those rags tight, into tight knots . . .

Proud of the good work you are doing . . .

Feeling good about yourself . . .

Again, you may not be a rug braider, so it is important to select some replacement behaviors that make sense for you. Some of these behaviors are listed in Chapter 17 and they range from handicrafts to housekeeping, and they work! You can sublimate eating from frustration into creative behavior.

Feel the deep sense of satisfaction about yourself . . .

See yourself in your bedroom chair . . .

See the vivid colors of the rug . . .

See the wonderful object you are creating . . .

And you feel very good about yourself . . .

Strong and confident, now that you do not rush to the kitchen . . .

Feeling very exhilarated and pleased with yourself . . .

Now . . .

At the count of three you are going to wake up feeling very refreshed . . .

Deeply relaxed . . .

Feeling wonderful . . .

Full of positive feelings . . .

Full of energy for the evening ahead . . .

One . . .

Two . . .

Three . . .

Eyes open . . .

Feeling wonderful . . .

Feeling relaxed . . .

You will find that this script will enable you to deal with the frustration you feel in domestic conflict situations and in other conflict situations that create a feeling of frustration that has resulted in abusing food or drink.

Furthermore, although no attempt is made herein to deal with particular domestic conflict situations—of which there are many—you will find that the relaxing effect of this evening tape and the reduction of the principal attitudes that cause food and drink abuse (hostility, anxiety, guilt, self-pity, self-punishment, depression) will in fact help communication between you and your domestic partner. You will find that in fact you do not anger as easily, and that discussions of subjects that previously led quickly to warfare may resolve themselves more readily. As you become calm and at peace with yourself, this feeling is sensed by your partner, and he may "get off his high horse" or "out of his tree," and the domestic tranquility will improve.

Maybe he will even try **TAPING IT OFF!**

CHAPTER THIRTEEN

MY ENEMIES, THE CHILDREN

For many parents—and not only mothers!—the stress of raising children in many of their growing-up years is one long conflict situation seeming to require generous overeating and overdrinking.

Children can create gigantic feelings of worry and anxiety, both of which we have seen as principal producers of poor eating and drinking behavior. Those little sweethearts are also capable of creating in parents large feelings of self-pity and "look-what-I've-given-up-for-you!"—also strong motivators of a run to the refrigerator. If your children (or whomever, for that matter) won't give you the respect and recognition you so richly deserve, why, then, there's always the kitchen.

Let's imagine that you are the mother of a 14-year-old daughter who has just returned from a day's classes at the high school with the brand new (and very expensive) jacket that you bought on sale stuffed into her backpack. Let us further imagine that you asked her why her jacket, on this chilly October day, was in her backpack rather than on her. And finally, let us postulate that she screams at you that she never liked the jacket anyway and never intended to wear it and wouldn't wear it to a dog fight, and storms into her room and slams the door.

Let us imagine that your 14-year-old son has gone surfing with the assurance to you that he "will be back before long," and it's 8:30 in the evening, has been dark for two hours, and the waves look awfully stormy and dark to you. (Of course no one wants to go surfing when the waves are calm!) Or let's suppose your older daughter, who was supposed to be home with her date at midnight, is still not home and it is 2:15. Let's further suppose that her date, who claims to be a 20-year-old, looks like he's 26, and the high school ballgame couldn't have lasted beyond 10 PM.

Or let us suppose that your youngest son, on his first report card, hasn't received a single grade better than a C−. Let's further suppose that he says every night at the dinner table—not unreasonably—that he hates school, and that the life of a merchant seaman seems thrilling for him.

Beginning to feel a little hungry? (Or maybe a couple of glasses of wine . . .)

This post-hyp script will prepare you to deal with the feelings of anxiety, anger, and frustration caused by those dearest of our enemies, our children. And if there's one guiding phrase in this script it is the following: It's going to be all right!

In a low monotone, tape the following suggestions and play them back to yourself, following your induction script.

You are very relaxed . . .

Ten minutes of time will seem like a single minute to you . . .

Time will go very very quickly . . .

Seeming like an instant . . .

And in less than an hour you can accomplish an entire day's work and do it more effectively than you normally would.

Now see yourself sitting on the bank of a river . . .

Looking up at a tree . . .

On which you see a bluebird . . .

It is springtime . . .

Smell the freshness in the air and the smell of honeysuckle . . .

Now the bird has flown from the branch and is flying toward you . . .

Hear the splashing of the river as the water falls in the rapids . . .

The bluebird is coming closer . . .

Look up the river, and at the end see a pink castle with flags waving from its turrets . . .

The bird is getting much closer . . .

A breeze blows out of the woods bringing the smell of ham from a picnic lunch that is spread before you on a checkered cloth . . .

You see ham, French bread, cheese, and wine . . .

Notice the pattern on the red and white checks on the spread . . .

You feel a feather brush against your hand, tickling your skin.

Now you feel the weight and heat of the bluebird as it lights on your hand . . .

You look into the eyes of the bird . . .

You see in his eyes the reflection of yourself . . .

Trim and attractive . . .

Sitting under a tree by the river . . .

You are surrounded by patches of white and yellow daisies . . .

You are a beautiful part of the environment . . .

Now the tree becomes transparent, and turns to glass . . .

Hanging from its branches are long loops of a glittery moss-like substance . . .

Now the bird closes his eyes . . .

Now the scene is gone . . .

You have now deepened your relaxation and practiced producing time condensation. Your ability to shorten your perception of "bad times" occasioned by conflict with your children will be very helpful in producing good eating behavior.

Now we are going to describe a typical parent-child conflict situation, and you will see yourself dealing with this problem in a positive manner. Obviously you must, when you write your own script in Chapter 18, outline an existing problem that is real for you. *In our example we'll use a mother-daughter conflict over kitchen clean-up—but the same principles can be used in any teen-age rebellion situation.*

(For the best ways to deal with teen-age children, we commend you to other books and/or your own conscience!)

See your daughter hurrying out of the kitchen, on her way to her room . . .

Where she will close the door and turn on the radio . . .

See the bread and peanut butter jar with the top still off . . .

See the knife and the smeared peanut butter on the counter . . .

Again, use the facts of your own situation. It may not be peanut butter! (You may wish it were peanut butter!)

Now see yourself walking to your daughter's room . . .

Knocking on the door . . .

Continuing to knock, knowing she hears you even with the radio turned up . . .

Seeing yourself at the point where you usually become furious . . .

And now seeing yourself from the outside . . .

As though you were an angel, hovering above the scene . . .

Seeing yourself calm and positive . . .

But very firm . . .

An adult cannot be baited by childish behavior . . .

Seeing yourself floating above the anger you feel . . .

Feeling firm . . .

And feeling very good about yourself . . .

Now your daughter is opening the door, with a very truculent look on her face . . .

There is that irritable, ready-to-fight look on her face . . .

Ready to mock you . . .

That look you know so well . . .

Now you see yourself telling her in as few words as you can what restrictions or additional duties she will incur by not cleaning up the kitchen when she is through . . .

By not speaking politely . . .

You see yourself looking her in the eye . . .

With a quiet firmness . . .

And you see yourself not rising to the scornful remark she makes . . .

Now you see yourself going upstairs . . .

Feeling good about your firmness . . .

Feeling good that you did not let her draw you into an angry argument . . .

But feeling full of energy and purpose . . .

Working your anger out in a constructive way . . .

Instead of going right back into the kitchen and cleaning up the peanut butter yourself—perhaps having some of it to make yourself feel better!—you will now suggest an image to yourself of doing one of the "replacement behaviors" outlined in greater detail in Chapter 17.

Now you see yourself going to your macrame basket . . .

Picking up the fibers . . .

Feeling how good the rope feels to your fingers . . .

Feeling its texture . . .

And seeing yourself begin to plait a new strand . . .

Feeling soothed by the activity . . .

Feeling very satisfied . . .

Letting the anger drain out of your fingertips . . .

Feeling the angry thoughts expressing themselves in your mind . . .

And draining down through your arms . . .

And out your fingers . . .

Feeling much better . . .

In knowing that your daughter will learn . . .

That she is a good girl . . .

And that she is going to turn out all right . . .

You are now comfortable with confronting her . . .

Setting limits . . .

And giving her the consequences if she oversteps those limits . . .

You are feeling very serene and happy . . .

And tomorrow morning . . .

When she is just waking up . . .

You will give her a hug and a kiss . . .

Now, at the count of three you are going to wake up feeling very refreshed . . .

Deeply relaxed . . .

Feeling wonderful . . .

Full of energy and positive feelings for the evening ahead . . .

One . . .

Two . . .

Three . . .

Eyes opened . . .

Feeling wonderful . . .

Feeling relaxed . . .

It's hard, when children are going through what seems to be a continuous and endless rebellion, to keep a calm and positive attitude as a parent. This tape will help you achieve that state of mind so that you can enjoy your children during their rough passage through adolescence!

CHAPTER FOURTEEN

NIGHTTIME NOSHING

Boredom is one of the great reasons for eating.

And although boredom is not limited to evenings, a repetitive theme in overweight patients is that of post-prandial snacking—or even gorging, in some cases.

Nighttime noshing takes two different major forms: the "snack before retiring" and "tube fodder." In the first instance there is at least the benefit of some slight common sense. After all, you haven't had anything to eat for four or five hours and you're getting a little hungry. In this instance you simply need to be sure that you are eating the correct small snack before going to bed and not giving yourself another full meal.

The more common problem behavior is that of a person watching television the whole evening and getting that bowl of buttered popcorn, followed by the dessert, to help along the plots of the television shows being watched. As the evening drones on, what better way to get a little excitement than to feed your face?!

The nature of television itself is such that you find yourself truly being a *spectator.* The camera makes you a little bit like a Peeping Tom, peeking into the living room of the characters of the situation comedy or the panelists on the *Tonight Show.* Perhaps one of the reasons for the popularity of news programming is that the anchor people seem to be speaking directly to you, and the news footage to some degree seems to put you near the action—but even the news shows have the characteristic, at best, of a lecture. You are being talked to, all right, but you are not being asked to talk *back*—at least to the network people! (People watching news shows, I'm convinced, vent more emotions to other people in the room than they do while watching any other type of show, with the possible exception of sports programs.)

But let's not leave too much at television's doorstep. If the set is broken and down at the repair shop, it is perfectly possible to have a bowl of popcorn while you are staring at the wall.

The point is that in the evenings you must learn to do something that relaxes you, gives you satisfaction, and probably involves your hands. Using your hands to do something besides feeding your face is the key to coping with nighttime boredom. These activities are dealt with in some detail in Chapter 17, "Replacement Behaviors."

In this post-hyp script, you will learn to transfer feelings of heat and dryness, which will demonstrate again to you that you can control the false feelings of hunger that drive you to the refrigerator. You will also give yourself adverse instructions about entering the kitchen in the evening.

In a low monotone, read the following script onto your tape after the induction script.

You are very, very cold. It is 20° below zero and all you can see is a bright blue and blinding white. Banks of white snow and sheets of shining ice. You are at the polar ice cap at the North Pole. The sky is so blue it almost hurts to look at it, and the sun is a cold, pale yellow.

You are tramping through the snow. You see the mouth of a cavern, and all around this cavern are long icicles sparkling in the sun. You walk up to the cavern, taking the glove off your right hand, and grab an icicle. The heat from your hand begins to melt the ice. You run your hand up and down the cold . . . wet . . . surface of the icicle. Now you put your glove back on.

Now you walk into the cave, and in the center of the cave is a large lake of ice cold water, dark and deep. You take a tin cup from your pack, and scoop up a cup of water, bringing the cold . . . dry metal of the cup to your lips . . .

feeling the cold liquid pouring down your throat into your stomach . . .

feeling the cold radiating from the center of your body.

Now you walk back to the mouth of the cave, your footsteps echoing off the cavern walls. As you stand looking at the blinding white snow, you hear a loud beating of mechanical wings. You look up and see a helicopter. A cold wind is created by the helicopter blades as it comes down to you and lands. You walk to the helicopter, and take the glove from your right hand. You put your right hand on the hot . . . dry . . . metal of the helicopter near the engine. When you feel that dry heat in your hand, you place your right hand on your right cheek . . .

Now let the dry heat in your right hand drain into your cheek . . .

Your cheek is becoming hot and flushed . . .

The blood is running to the surface of the skin . . .

It feels as if hot air is blowing against it . . .

Now your hand is becoming cold. When all the heat has drained from your hand into your cheek, you once again place your hand at your side.

Now you once again place your right hand on your right cheek. Let the dry . . . warmth . . . in your cheek drain back into your hand. When all that warmth has drained from your cheek back into your hand, you once again place your hand at your side. You find your hand becoming hot and dry . . . and your cheek is becoming cool.

You will quickly see that these sensations that you call hunger and emptiness are mental attitudes, and you can control them easily by learning the skills to do so. There is nothing complicated or difficult about this: You simply learn to "close off" these sensations or to transfer them to another part of your body.

You get into the helicopter. You fasten your seatbelt, and feel its pressure around your middle as the helicopter begins to lift off the ground. You are surrounded by a silver mist as you go higher . . . and higher . . . and higher . . .

You look at the altitude gauge and see you are five thousand feet in the air . . .

And now you go back to 2,000 feet above sea level, where you land.

In front of you on a plate is a hot, fragrant steak, and a bowl of crisp green salad. You start eating the steak . . .

And its flavor is all the good things you have ever remembered about eating steak . . .

It is delicious . . .

Now you see yourself eating the salad . . .

Eating slowly . . .

And you keep eating until your stomach begins to swell . . .

You see the difference between the pressure on the inside of your stomach from the food you were eating . . .

And the pressure on the outside of your stomach from the seatbelt of the helicopter . . .

Feel the difference . . .

Now the helicopter is beginning to descend. You feel that sinking feeling in the pit of your stomach . . .

Five thousand feet . . .

Four thousand feet . . .

Three thousand feet . . .

Two thousand feet . . .

One thousand feet.

This is very odd. You were to land at two thousand feet above sea level, but the helicopter continues to go down . . .

As the plane goes lower . . .

And lower . . .

It gets hotter and hotter inside the compartment. At one thousand feet it is 80°. . .

And at sea level it is 90° above zero . . .

And now you are at minus one thousand feet according to the altimeter and it is 100° in the cabin . . .

At minus two thousand feet it is 110° in the cabin. At three thousand feet below sea level the helicopter lands.

Perspiration is streaming down your forehead and your armpits . . .

Your clothes are stuck to your body . . .

And the inside of the compartment is steamed up . . .

Your hair is matted to your forehead, and it is very stuffy.

Then you open the door and get out. In front of you is the world as it was millions of years ago . . .

A deep, thick, steamy forest, with huge redwoods and enormous ferns—a thick jungle with gigantic old trees. You walk over to a river of boiling water.

You hold your hand above the boiling water and feel the hot . . . wet steam collecting on the palm of your right hand. When you feel this wet heat on your right hand, place your right hand on your right cheek . . .

And let that wet heat . . .

Drain into your cheek. The cheek is getting wet and hot and sweaty . . .

And your hand becomes cool as if being held in front of a fan.

When all the wet heat has drained from your hand into your cheek, you once again place your right hand at your side. Now once again put your right hand on your right cheek, and let that wet heat in your cheek drain back into your hand. When all the wet heat in your cheek is drained back into your hand, once again put your hand at your side. Your cheek is becoming cool and dry . . .

And your hand is moist and hot as if it is being held over a kettle steaming on the stove.

Now you lie down beside the river in the forest, and you smell wet earth underneath you, drifting off in a world that existed millions of years ago . . .

Drifting and floating . . .

Relaxing very deeply . . .

Dreaming . . .

Feeling wonderful.

This completes the deepening section of your script, and you'll now give youself some specific instructions to deal with nighttime noshing.

You see yourself sitting there in the chair, watching television on an evening . . .

An evening with no favorite shows . . .

Nothing you have been looking forward to seeing . . .

But watching television anyway, trying to find something to fill up the time . . .

And you find yourself thinking that a bowl of hot, buttered popcorn would taste good . . .

Again, use here specific foods that you commonly eat in the evening after dinner, whether it be candy, ice cream, cookies, or potato chips.

But when this thought comes to you, you immediately think of your new behavior in the evening, and the pleasure it gives you.

In Chapter 17 there are many, many replacement behaviors given to suggest to you possible activities for your hands when you are bored. At this point you would select one or more of these activities and give yourself an instruction to think of this activity rather than going to the refrigerator. For purposes of illustration, we will use crewel, the loosely twisted yarn used for embroidery.

You find yourself picking up the crewel pattern of the beautiful colors illustrating the lake and trees . . .

Finding yourself deeply soothed and deeply contented with the satisfaction you are gaining from completing this beautiful pattern . . .

Knowing that people will praise your skill . . .

And that it will make your home even more beautiful . . .

The selection of the kinds of handicraft or placement activity is very important, since you are tired in the evenings, and you need to find an activity that is satisfying yet not creating more tension, and thereby creating a greater need for food and drink. Some people are able to find the energy and satisfaction in restoring old homes in the evenings—but many will find they need a more relaxing activity.

Feel the satisfaction and relaxation flow through your body as you undertake a new section of the pattern . . .

Enjoying the colors of the work . . .

And the texture of the yarn . . .

Feeling deeply pleased . . .

Now you will see the refrigerator door in your kitchen . . .

And the cupboard where your foodstuffs are kept . . .

And you'll see that they are not to be opened during the evening . . .

After dinner . . .

And if you go to the refrigerator or the cupboard door . . .

You will notice that it is very hard to open . . .

And when you touch this door in the evening . . .

This action will remind you to turn around and go back into the other room . . .

Picture and describe your particular refrigerator here in great detail. Mention its pattern and color and shape of its handle.

Now, at the count of three you're going to wake up feeling very fresh . . .

Deeply relaxed . . .

Feeling wonderful and full of energy . . .

Hold positive thoughts for the evening ahead . . .

One . . .

Two . . .

Three . . .

Eyes open! . . .

Feeling wonderful and feeling relaxed.

You will find that this particular problem eating behavior, if it is one that troubles you, is one of the quickest to correct using the power of self-instruction contained in this book. And the double benefit of putting replacement behaviors in place is that you will be creating some new beauty of your own while you're recreating yourself! These new habits will result in a much better looking body, of course, but they will also result in a healthier body, enabling you to live a longer and more satisfying life.

There is no reason at all that this won't work for you, and you simply need fifteen minutes a day to *TAPE IT OFF!*

CHAPTER FIFTEEN

I WISH I WERE PREGNANT

The lack of love—or human fulfillment—is something we all feel at times, and it's something felt by both men and women. When this feeling becomes a persistent one, it is often described as a "feeling of emptiness," and is often expressed as a lack of someone who loves you, or in a larger sense, a loss of a sense of purpose in your life. (Hence the title for this chapter, since for people of a certain age, pregnancy may seem to fill this void for a temporary period of time. Unfortunately, pregnancy usually causes its own reasons to overeat!)

Eating and drinking are very basic and almost simpleminded ways that people use to try to fill this described "emptiness."

In this script you will focus on seeing yourself engaging in behaviors that interact with other people, and with social or personal activities that seem important to you—whether they be the care of lost cats or campaigning for political candidates.

You will make a list of the things you really care about. What do you like to do? Suppose you found yourself at a time when money was not a factor: You are "well to do" in a time in your life with no family responsibilities, and no one to tell you what you *should* do or what was appropriate for you to do.

What, then, would you do for the *satisfaction* of it? Make a list of these things, because you are going to use them in this tape if you find yourself with the problem of overeating and overdrinking to sooth this vague restlessness or emptiness that keeps coming to your mind.

And remember, it keeps coming to your *mind.* Your mind is the instrument of your satisfaction, or of your downfall. It isn't too much to say that "you weigh what you think." But fortunately, attitudes can be changed and you're just the person to change them!

Read the following script to yourself in a low monotone following an induction script. The first part of this script will deepen your relaxation state, and give you a set of images to produce greater control over your physical functioning.

You are in a huge meadow with a vast expanse of blue sky above you. Spring is in the air, and you can smell its freshness. In the distance you can see the snow covered mountains, like the Alps in Austria. The meadow is green and covered with white daisies and bright blue wildflowers. You feel marvelous, and wish to climb to the top of the mountains.

You take a compressed air pump and place a rubber hose in your mouth, and then you begin pumping your body with air. . . . filling up like a balloon.

The light . . . dry . . . air gives you a feeling of weightlessness.

You begin to float up slowly into the blue sky . . .

Floating up . . .

And you are approaching the peaks of the mountain. You are getting much colder as you go up higher in the air . . .

As the altitude increases. The cold causes the air inside you to contract, and you begin to descend . . .

Landing on the ridge of the mountain top. You are freezing cold. The wind is blowing bitterly. With your back to the side of the mountain, you inch your way along the ledge as the cold snow blows in your face.

You come to a pass, and on the other side of the pass you find a whole different world. Suddenly you find yourself in a peach orchard. It is warm, like the middle of the summer, and the smell of the peaches is fragrant in the air, like a perfume. You see fountains and marble statues. One statue looks like you—slim and supple and light of foot in its pose. You touch the statue and feel the smoothness of its alabaster.

Passing through the orchard, you come to a long flight of stone stairs leading up to a palace cut from rocks. Slowly you walk up the steps . . .

Up the steps . . .

Into the temple . . .

Finding yourself in a large chamber.

You see before you a long trestle table on which is a plate with a stack of steaming pancakes covered with butter and syrup. Next to them is a pitcher of milk. You begin eating the pancakes, and gulping them down with milk. You feel starved. They taste delicious, and you eat and eat, shoving the food down as though you never would eat again.

At this point you are likely to find yourself salivating if you like pancakes! This is simply one more indication of the physical effects you can readily call up in yourself and another proof to you that you'll be able to give your body instructions to eat the kind of foods that will make it healthful and trim.

The pancake dough seems to be getting heavier and heavier in the pit of your stomach, weighting you down with a wet. . . .heavy. . . .mass. Your stomach feels enormously heavy, as though there were a lead ball inside it . . .

So heavy now that you cannot even stand up . . .

Suddenly a gong sounds, echoing throughout the chamber . . .

And a sliding stone door opens. A very old man with a wispy beard comes in, bringing a foaming glass of pink liquid. You realize it is an ancient health drink, containing yeast. The old man gives it to you and you drink.

Now you feel the yeast inside your stomach making bubbles, making you feel lighter and lighter and lighter . . .

Light . . .

with . . .

bubbles inside you make you feel as light as a feather. You float along the floor as if there were no gravity . . .

As if you were an astronaut. You cannot keep your feet on the floor, because you are feeling so light.

You glide along the floor, out the door of the rock palace . . .

Floating down the steps, touching every fourth one lightly with a toe . . .

And float to a nearby river.

You float like an innertube in the river to the exact place that you entered the peach orchard, smelling once again the delightful, warm fragrance of the peaches and their ripeness. You are once again at the entry to the orchard.

Immediately you feel a great heaviness in your bones . . .

You have dry . . .

Heavy bones.

They weigh down your arms and legs as though these bones were made from the heaviest of lead. You lie down in the orchard where you entered, but you can hear the sound of the howling wind outside on the cold mountain ridge. You are getting very sleepy indeed.

So sleepy . . .

Feeling relaxed . . .

Wonderful . . .

In complete control of your appetites.

You have, by this point, experienced several sensations in your body relating to eating and drinking. More importantly, you have seen how you can call up the "sensations" of hunger, and how readily you can call up the feelings of satiation, heaviness, dryness, and other physical sensations in your body. You now know that you can recall these feelings whenever you need to, and whenever they will help you eliminate the need to overeat or drink.

Now you are going to use one of the activities that you really would like to do in your script, and see yourself doing it.

For the purposes of this illustration, we will presume that you have always wanted to teach young children swimming, and that you enjoy the activity of swimming. Whatever the activity, it should be important to you. *If the activity is one that makes you move your body around—whether it be walking door to door getting petitions signed for a political cause, or teaching swimming to youngsters—so much the better! Exercise is valuable to your body, but it's probably more valuable to your mind: When you are moving around, the organs work properly and keep the mind alert, and occupied with something other than "emptiness."*

You feel the splash of the water and hear the laughter of the children . . .

Feeling their slick, wet arms and legs . . .

Laughing yourself as they splash you with water . . .

Hearing the sound of their happy laughter echo in the enclosed pool . . .

Hearing yourself laugh . . .

Feeling a part of the laughter . . .

Seeing the progress of the little boy who used to sink to the bottom of the pool like a stone . . .

Seeing the thankfulness in his pride in his eyes . . .

And knowing the gratefulness he feels toward you . . .

Seeing the young girls blossom with self-confidence as their swimming improves . . .

Seeing the healthy relationships develop between the young boys and girls . . .

And feeling very proud that you are such a part of their lives . . .

Giving them strength and the mental attitudes to deal with life's difficulties . . .

Feeling yourself strong and calm with an infinite strength to give . . .

Seeing them crowding around you . . .

Touching you . . .

Hugging you . . .

Laughing.

Knowing that you are making a difference with your life and its activities . . .

And knowing that your life is very important.

Feeling very strong and secure and full of purpose.

Feeling wonderful.

Now at the count of three you're going to wake up feeling very refreshed . . .

Deeply relaxed . . .

Feeling wonderful . . .

Full of energy . . .

Full of positive feelings for the evening ahead . . .

One . . .

Two . . .

Three!

Eyes open . . .

Feeling wonderful . . .

And feeling deeply relaxed and full of energy.

Life is full of many activities that are pleasurable, and you will have no trouble finding some that suit you and replace your overeating and overdrinking. There are so many enjoyable and satisfying things to do!

You are going to have a marvelous new life, and you will find that excess weight drops off almost mysteriously as you correct the reasons for your eating and drinking abuse. Just *TAPE IT OFF!* every day for fifteen minutes!

CHAPTER SIXTEEN

DRINKING AGAIN

Abuse of alcohol is a behavior problem of its own, and deserves more than a single chapter to treat the problem in all its dimensions. However, for many people with an alcohol or drug abuse problem, the profoundly relaxing effect of fifteen minutes spent each evening listening to the induction and post-hypnotic tape can provide the attitude restructuring and relaxation and anxiety reduction necessary to change their lives.

Drinking, in relation to obesity and fatness, is not the principal cause of excess poundage. But any weight reduction program that ignores overdrinking leaves a big loophole, since liquor contains additional calories, and these calories go down so readily! Besides the "sneaky" addition of these calories to your diet, liquor produces a relaxed, devil-may-care attitude toward eating, thereby vastly multiplying the number of calories already taken in.

The alcoholic personality often encountered exhibits many of these character traits: over-sensitivity, feelings of inadequacy and lack of self esteem, inability to tolerate frustration well, deep feelings (often repressed) of hostility, exaggerated capacity for self-pity, often over-protected as a child, and frequently a connoisseur of the injustices of life.

Given this set of doleful attitudes, it isn't surprising to find that alcohol relieves the tension that this person feels, and "makes him/her feel better."

What may be surprising is to find that the daily fifteen minutes of deep relaxation that your tape produces—and the replacement behaviors with their feelings of deep satisfaction and accomplishment—also relieves these feelings of the alcoholic personality. For the severe alcoholic personality, of course, professional treatment is required, but these same principles will be employed: In the short term change the symptoms (the drinking), and in the long term change the causes *(attitudes and feelings)*.

In this chapter you will learn to give yourself instructions that will change your alcohol abuse by adverse pairing. You will also learn to avoid habitual geographic customs like the corner bar or the liquor store.

Lest all this sound too depressing to you if you are one of the millions who enjoy alcohol, take heart!

You will, if you wish, be able to give yourself instructions to avoid alcohol on all occasions except Friday and Saturday evenings, for example, or on all occasions except parties, or some similar clear demarcation. Depending upon the degree of your alcohol dependency and personality traits, you *may* (emphasize *may*) be able to give yourself instructions limiting yourself to a single glass of wine in the evening.

But during any attempt to lose weight this is not advisable. Wait for four or five months, when your eating and drinking habits have been restructured, and then consider how one or two drinks in the evening—*carefully measured!*— will fit into your weight maintenance of the new, trim, slim you.

You will find yourself happily surprised that the deeply relaxing evening tape does a better job than booze!

In a low monotone read the following script onto your tape following the induction script you select.

You are on a fishing boat in the Bahamas, and the day is warm, the sky is a vivid blue, achingly blue. The sun is almost white in the sky. The shore, as you sit in the boat, is lined with bright white sand and palm trees, and perspiration sits on your skin. Brilliant colored flowers line the coast.

You are wearing scuba diving gear with an oxygen tank on your back. You are sitting on the edge of the boat ready to fall into the warm water and dive. Feel your body falling backwards . . .

Somersaulting backwards into the warm water . . .

Going around and around . . .

Head over heels into the warm tropical water . . .

As you go deeper . . .

Deeper . . .

And deeper . . .

The water gets cooler and cooler.

As you go deeper and deeper it gets darker . . .

Darker.

You see bright salmon-colored coral and fan-shaped plants, and fish with many colors on their scales. You see bright goldfish and lime-green fish and orange angel fish catching rays of sunlight as they dart quickly by.

Now you see a cold, blue object that looks like a net. You approach it and touch it. It sends a terrific jolt of electricity through your whole body. It feels as if you have touched an electric wire or put your finger in a light socket. But the feeling is pleasant . . .

Very stimulating . . .

Like a light electrical charge running through your bones and making them *hot* . . .

And dry.

Once again you are learning to control your body's reaction to your suggestions as to how you can feel and to how it will react to the food and drink that you are going to put into it.

As you continue to go deeper, you get colder and colder. You become encased in a huge block of ice. Your skin and your body parts are numb . . .

Like wood.

The block of ice with you frozen inside it bobs to the surface, and floats to the shore drifting on the water up onto the hot sand.

Your block of ice, with you still in it, melts in the strong heat of the white hot sun. Your muscles feel like jelly as they thaw out and the heat rushes back into them. But your bones inside your muscles are still frozen solid . . .

Cold . . .

Dry . . .

Your blood is cold like ice water . . .

Wet . . .

And cold in your body . . .

Forcing its way through your arteries and veins.

You begin to shiver with chills in the blazing tropic sun as the ice water runs through your veins . . .

And your skin surface is hot . . .

It is as though you have fever chills with influenza.

Suddenly your eye sees a bottle washed upon the shore. You go over to it. It is a bottle of whisky. You begin drinking.

What do you habitually drink? The type of alcoholic beverage should be used here if it is not, in fact, whisky.

See the label on the bottle. Feel the shape of the bottle in your hand.

Now you are drinking more. You are becoming intoxicated . .

And your head is beginning to spin as you try to walk. Your blood is hot . . .

Wet . . .

Feeling on fire in your veins. You lie down on the hot sand . . .

And all the vivid colors of the flowers and the sky around you begin to swirl and become molten and blend together . . .

They are spinning around and around . . .

You feel yourself whirling and spinning . . .

Seeing liquid purples and greens and reds and gold blending together . . .

Spinning . . .

Spinning . . .

Now you are vomiting . . .

Deeply and thoroughly throwing up the whisky . . .

Expelling it . . .

Now you are lying down . . .

Completely calm . . .

Every muscle in your body relaxed . . .

Now that the whisky is out of your body . . .

Feeling extremely relaxed . . .

Content and satisfied . . .

Feeling very happy . . .

And sleeping.

You have just given yourself an adverse instruction. Now you are going to give yourself a positive image. You should imagine yourself in a typical drinking situation, wherever that may be. Do you drink in your living room or at a bar with friends? You must write this scene in your own script using all of your five senses of taste, smell, hearing, sight, and touch. For purposes of this script we are going to assume that you drink in your living room.

You are in your living room in the evening . . .

Sitting in your favorite chair . . .

Feeling the worn spot on the arm . . .

And the pleasant pressure of the seat cushion . . .

Smelling the smoke of the oak fire burning gently in the fireplace . . .

Seeing the soft glow of the table lamp falling on the polished oak end table . . .

Hearing the gentle popping of the fire, burning in the fireplace just before needing a fresh log . . .

Tasting the fresh carrot you have just chewed . . .

With its optimistic flavor . . .

Now you see a glass of whisky on the table . . .

See your hand reaching out for it . . .

Picking it up and smelling it . . .

Smell the rich, marvelous smell . . .

Come and see yourself put it back on its coaster . . .

The little straw coaster with the green stripes . . .

Putting the cold glass down on the coaster . . .

And seeing your hand come away from the glass.

Now remember your deep relaxation on the beach in the Bahamas . . .

Feel how deeply relaxed you were after expelling all that whisky . . .

Lying on the beach . . .

Feeling marvelous.

Now you see yourself reaching for the glass again . . .

But stopping before you touch the glass . . .

And now you remember once again the marvelous feelings you had on the beach in the Bahamas when you got this awful whisky out of your body . . .

Finally, you're going to go beyond sensory recall to emotional recall. You will use this "peak experience" imaging in your final "write your own script" chapter. Practice it here. Remember a time in your life when you felt the exhilaration and elation of accomplishment. Maybe you had a moment of triumph at work; maybe it was a personal or sexual moment. Remember it vividly and see yourself doing it. See yourself reliving it. For purposes of illustration in this script, we will assume this moment to be the moment you were elected class president in high school.

As you see your hand coming away from the glass, you recall the elation and exhilaration when they announced your name in the school auditorium as the winner in the race to be senior class president . . .

Feel it now . . .

Feel the elation!

Feel the exhilaration and power surge through your body as a result of declining to drink this whisky . . .

Feeling marvelous in your judgment and what you elect to do with your time . . .

And your self-discipline . . .

And the feeling that you are in charge of your life . . .

This section of the script that follows is optional. *It is a much more strongly adverse set of instructions to yourself, and should be used only if needed. Generally it is preferable to deal with restructuring your attitudes with positive imagery, as too much negative imagery can create tension, which is what you are trying to decrease.*

Now imagine yourself riding in an airplane. Feel the motion of the plane as it bounces around the sky. Look out the window. See the bright blue sky and the white fluffy clouds. You are drinking whisky over ice. Taste it. Roll it on your tongue. Smell it, both with your nose and with your mouth through your nasal passages. Smell and taste the strong flavor and smell.

Suddenly the man sitting next to you bends over and vomits. Smell the vomit. The sour smell of his vomit is all over you. There are pieces of this vomit in your drink. Green and yellow slime is running down your glass.

You take another gulp of your whisky, and see chunks of his vomit sloshing together with the whisky. Pieces of this vomit catch in your throat, but you keep drinking.

A stronger feeling of nausea and sickness is coming over you with each gulp you take. Your stomach is swelling and distending from all the alcohol you are drinking. You are licking the slime from the rim of your glass, until finally . . .

You retch and begin vomiting yourself. Vomit and whisky are all over, and the plane is lurching and bouncing around in the sky . . .

Dipping like a roller coaster . . .

Bouncing around in the turbulent weather it has encountered.

From this day on, whenever you taste or smell whisky . . .

You will think of this vomit and nausea and air sickness.

The above text should be particularized to your own personal experiences. If you were ever badly seasick, describe this fact to yourself in some great detail rather than using an airplane. Use a memorable personal experience of nausea, and describe the detail of its occurrence using all five of your senses. You will give yourself instructions for some replacement behavior that will make you feel satisfied and worthwhile as a person. Select a replacement behavior from Chapter 17. The example below will once again use crewel, a form of needlework.

Now see yourself pulling yarn through the pattern . . .

Creating a beautiful picture of an owl in a barn . . .

See the browns and greys . . .

Feel the soft yarn and the rough texture of the pattern in your hand . . .

Think how attractive this will be . . .

Of the compliments you will get . . .

Think of the value you have as a person . . .

And feel elated and deeply contented . . .

Now at the count of three you are going to wake up feeling very refreshed . . .

Deeply relaxed . . .

Feeling wonderful and full of energy . . .

Full of positive feelings for the evening ahead and the next day . . .

One . . .

Two . . .

Three . . .

Eyes open! . . .

Feeling wonderful . . .

Feeling relaxed.

CHAPTER SEVENTEEN

REPLACEMENT BEHAVIORS

This chapter will help you undertake activities that are fun and satisfying and that will replace your need to rush to the refrigerator.

Let's take a moment to consider what kind of behavior you are trying to replace. By now, you should be able to write down your "problem times." When does your overeating (and/or overdrinking) take place? What time of day? Where does it take place? What rooms in your house or what physical location? Identify these problem times and write them on a piece of paper. They are not mysterious; they are well known to you.

For a significant number of people these behavior problems will center in the evening after dinner, but whatever time of the day and whatever place you are having your problems with boredom, frustration, anger, anxiety, and other emotions that are inducing you to eat, consider this:

You eat with your hands. (Or at least we certainly hope so!)

So at one level you need to find some replacement activities that occupy your hands, and as luck would have it, there are dozens of handicraft activities that fill this bill very nicely.

On another level, it is important to find an activity that is mentally refreshing or soothing. While you would undoubtedly find many handicrafts requiring careful and close work that would fulfill the need to occupy your hands, if you are not skilled at fine and close work with your hands this activity would simply create a tension and anxiety level that would send you right back to the refrigerator. So you need to try a number of handicrafts to find one which is satisfying to you.

A word of caution here: Find a handicraft which is satisfying to you *in and of itself*. You are not doing these handicrafts for the admiration of others, or as examples of your artistry to be praised and evaluated. You are doing it for the pleasure of the activity itself, and the soothing effect it has. If your friends and family like and praise the outcome of your work, fine. *But this is not the purpose of the activity*. You are not undertaking this with the thought of becoming a great artist; if it works out that way, fine.

Think of the paintings by Winston Churchill, who undertook the activity as a relaxation. A psychiatrist of my acquaintance does pillow embroidery as he sits listening to patients, helping them work their way through the problems of life.

It's also important for you to choose a handicraft that can be worked at continuously for a few minutes or a few hours, but not something that must be completed immediately. Once again, you are choosing a handicraft to give you satisfaction, not to create more stress in your life.

In this listing and thumbnail description of various handicrafts and replacement behaviors that follow, you will see that most of these are of low cost. We have avoided suggesting handicrafts that have a high entry equipment cost because you should have the freedom to try several handicrafts and find some that give you pleasure without having an investment to protect.

You will be surprised how much fun you're going to have!

A SELECTION OF CRAFTS

Crayon work includes designs with oil pastel crayons, water soluble crayons, chalk pastel crayons, or fluorescent crayons on a variety of surfaces including newsprint, heavy paper, cloth, and sandpaper. Designs can be done to your own liking through free hand or stencil.

Fresco is wall painting with water mixed colors on wet plaster.

Clay work takes in a wide range of possible crafts you can enjoy, getting at its most simple with coil building, slab cutting, and hollowing-out from solid balls of clay. Clay that hardens itself naturally can be purchased, and you can fire or glaze these objects later in a community kiln.

Ceramics is a more advanced form of clay work, and objects can be formed by pinch-forming, or using molds. To learn "throwing" objects using a wheel, you must take some adult education courses at your local high school or community college.

Mosaics comes from the Greek word which means "belonging to the muses," and is composed of small pieces of different colored material, called tesserae. This is a particularly relaxing hobby for many people.

Sculpture in clay media is a good way to explore this form, including direct modeling in terra cotta, modeling with an oil-based clay, modeling using an armature, and plaster casting.

Batik is a form of fabric design using dyes and wax to resist dyes. Additional designs are available or you can create your own.

Burlap can be made into lampshades, painted upon, embroidered, or stitched.

Felt crafting can include simple gluing of patterns on top of a brightly colored background, making stuffed dolls and animals, or making and framing felt flowers.

Macrame, another especially relaxing and occupying hobby for weight loss folks, consists of using a variety of knots on cords, twines, or yarns to make many useful objects from handbags to plant holders. One of its hidden qualities is that you may embark on an ambitious project with little advance planning, creating and changing design as you work. Macrame is also one of the least expensive crafts.

Needlecraft is one of the oldest crafts known, and encompasses embroidery, crewel (essentially embroidery with wool worsted yarns), applique, quilting, and needlepoint. Needless to say, each of these forms of needlecraft has its own extensive traditions and patterns.

Tie and dye is a simple technique to give fabrics such as drapes, shirts, pants, and umbrellas a fashionable look, and is fun to do.

Weaving can be undertaken with a small warp at home, and you can grow, as you enjoy the subject more, into larger looms as you discover if this is the craft for you.

Metal crafting is the art of making beautiful and useful objects from metals, especially these ten: gold, silver, copper, pewter, brass, bronze, nickel, silver, aluminum, and rod and cast iron.

Enameling is the fusing of glass colored with metallic oxides onto a metal surface, and can be used to make a wide variety of items from earrings and bowls to trays and boxes. Many pre-formed copper shapes are available from which to begin the enameling process. Specialized types of enameling are: cloisonne, which gives separation of enamel colors with wire barriers; and champleve, which uses etching of the metal and gives less precise separations.

Nail sculpture is a little-known and fascinating hobby involving bending and soldering nails—in particular, iron nails—into abstract designs for your walls and useful objects, such as candle holders and nameplates.

Repoussage, whose French name describes the easy craft of embossing on soft metals with special tools, requires only a minimum amount of equipment. Aluminum in thin sheets is the most common metal used for this—although copper, pewter, bronze, and brass are also possible—and your design is inscribed on soft metal that is placed on a hard rubber mat. An excellent aspect of this craft is that it can be done almost anywhere, even in a living room. The metal can be colored as well through a variety of techniques.

Stained glass can be cut and used for a fascinating variety of projects, including windows, lamps, pendants, and many other objects.

Tin can crafting enables you to cut, curl, arch, and bend these inexpensive and readily available materials into useful and decorative items.

Wire crafting can use almost any sort of wire from coat hangers to aluminum wire to silver and platinum, though most substantial craft projects use brass, copper, or steel wire. Depending upon the project, this again can be a good craft to do anywhere.

Lapidary, or gem cutting, uses more equipment than most of the crafts mentioned in this chapter, but can produce some beautiful stones for jewelry purposes. These stones can be found in gravel beds and excavations, and the stones need not be precious or semi-precious—they need merely be beautiful.

Paper craft includes a variety of techniques, such as weaving with paper, transparencies, mosaics, and the diorama.

Book binding can include gathering your favorite articles from particular magazines, season concert programs, or adding a hard and beautiful cover to your favorite paperback book.

Cardboard, especially reinforced or corrugated cardboard, makes a fine material for a variety of interesting objects from wastepaper baskets to dividers for drawers.

Coloring papers is a soothing and relaxing hobby that produces "designer papers" to use in wrapping presents and other uses. Techniques include wood stain coloring, water coloring, marbeling, felt tip work, and ink spraying.

Origami is the Japanese art of folding a single sheet of paper to resemble a multitude of objects without use of scissors or paste. A craft that travels well and makes delightful figures for children!

Scissors craft, as you would imagine, involves cutting intricate and pleasing shapes that can be mounted and framed for display. They can be used to make greeting cards or stationery, and the design will be your own. An inexpensive and convenient handicraft that you can take with you wherever you go!

Acrylic modeling paste and paint can be used to create forms and designs for cloth, sculpture, and collage. Easy and convenient.

Bead crafting is a craft as old as mankind, and one of the most soothing. You can create necklaces, bracelets, and wall designs.

Candle making is both useful and decorative. Candles can be made by rolling, dipping, multi-layering, and molding.

Leathercraft can provide you with everything from clothing to purses to boxes of great beauty and value. Stitching, cutting, and lacing are some of the hand skills needed.

Plastic foam can be used to make bathtub toys, bird houses, and many other durable objects. Tools needed include a sharp knife and a soldering gun with a flexible wire tip that can make deep "hot wire" cuts in foam, as well as an electrical woodburning pencil to bore holes. If you like this plastic foam work, you can at a later stage add a hot-wire cutter that rounds the edges while you cut.

Decoupage is the art of decorating with paper cutouts, having originated in Venice during the 17th century. Decoupage requires few tools and is extremely flexible. The paper cutouts can be applied to almost any surface, from wood and glass to metal and stone. Lamps, paperweights, papers, boxes, trays, and lampshades are only a few possibilities for the use of decoupage.

Mask-making can be used for creating wall decorations or gifts for children for Halloween and party purposes; types of masks include single folds, paper bag masks, papier mache, and chicken wire masks.

Matchbox crafting gives you the opportunity to make a variety of dollhouse furniture and little funny cars and automobiles.

Doll-making is one of the most relaxing and satisfying of handcrafts you can take up; you can create excellent and loving gifts for children and grandchildren. Dolls can be made from foam rubber, twigs, dowels—and can be modeled when you reach a stage of expertise to do this. Stuffed dolls have been popular for years with those who enjoy sewing, and the level of detail can easily be scaled to match your own preference, from large and loose to tiny and tight.

Wood carving and whittling allow you to turn plain objects into beautiful, ornamented works of art. Everything from bracelets and necklaces to carved figures and chess boards is possible!

IN SUM

You've only looked at a few of the possible handicrafts available to you to occupy your hands and your attention as a replacement activity for eating and drinking.

We have not even taken up whole areas of various art forms, including oil and acrylic painting, water colors, drawing, silk screening, intaglio, wood cutting, woodworking, and various printing processes. Many of these are taught in beginning and advanced courses at your local adult education department in high schools and community colleges, and from private crafts' people in your community.

Take a course and get out one or two days a week! Learn a new art or handicraft to occupy yourself!

Finally, when you have found a handicraft that you enjoy doing, instruct yourself in your tape to see yourself doing this particular handicraft, and feel the enjoyment you will receive from it. When you give yourself this positive instruction, you will find these replacement behaviors fitting well into your new, satisfying life. It is as though you took out an old, displeasing puzzle piece from the part of yourself causing difficulty, and replaced it with a new, pleasing piece. You will be astonished at how satisfying your new behavior will become to you.

Needless to say, the fact that you have replacement behaviors to drain off the stresses of everyday life will allow you not only to *TAPE IT OFF!*, but to *KEEP IT OFF!*

CHAPTER EIGHTEEN

A SCRIPT FOR YOU ONLY

Now you're going to put into action what you have read about in the last several chapters! You're going to change your attitudes about eating and drinking and lose the weight you want to lose safely, without drugs, and permanently!

The point has been made throughout that this script must be very personal and unique. It must relate to you, and to you only. No two people have exactly the same kitchens, and the very environments in which you have been eating and drinking incorrectly are critical to the attitude change you will achieve. Even if a husband and wife are undertaking this program at the same time, their tapes will be different because the personal histories of the two people will differ enough that the tapes should be tailored to their own histories. It is common, however, to see overlapping eating and drinking problems within the same families, so that large portions of the tape for members of the same family might well be used by two people.

ELEMENTS OF YOUR SCRIPT

Your first script and others you will write are made up basically of two sections: the induction section that puts you in what used to be called a trance state, and the deepening and post-hypnotic section, where you relax even more deeply and give yourself instructions for new attitudes based upon positive images and negative associations.

This book has given you many different scripts to serve as the basis for writing your own. Several induction scripts are given, as well as a wide variety of "post-hypnotic" scripts that deal with many common eating and drinking problems encountered by people who are overweight.

Now the question for you is this: Can you just pick an induction script and one of the post-hypnotic scripts and read them into a tape recorder?

Yes.

However, if you choose to do this, take special pains along the way, especially in your post-hypnotic script, to make the occasions of your bad eating and drinking unique to you. Put down exactly what it is you're eating and the place where you are overeating and drinking, and use little descriptions of the environment that will give you highly personal psychological "cues" to remind you of your new behavior.

Next, where replacement behaviors are called for—and they almost uniformly will be needed—use some of the replacement behavior suggested in Chapter 17 for your own personal script.

Again, this is an aspect of your tape that will be unique for you. No two people will have the same mixture of eating habits, eating environments, and replacement behaviors. You are a special person!

A WORD OF CAUTION

Fat, we emphasize again, is caused by six general behavior problems.

1. Too many meals and snacks and eating between meals.
2. Eating the wrong foods for the three meals a day you should eat.
3. Putting too much food on your plate.
4. Eating in the wrong environments (such as your living room while watching television).
5. Eating for emotional reasons (perhaps the most pervasive problem).
6. Not using enough energy for output or exercise.

Start with giving yourself instructions for reasons 1 and 4, and then add 5 and see how you're doing. If you start eating three meals a day, sitting down at a table, eating your meals slowly and chewing them well, you may find this is enough change in your behavior to lose weight.

If not, add instructions to yourself for your particular emotional eating problems. Remember positive times in your life and the many hopeful activities the world engages in. Use these as positive images to "bootstrap" your way out of negative feelings.

One strong image you can use when "wading in your swamp" is to see yourself climbing a short three-step ladder into a beautiful meadow filled with sunshine, and recall feelings of happiness and satisfaction that you have had in your life. This is a quick mood elevator.

There is an axiom in tennis which says: *Always change a losing game.* If your mental attitude is negative, don't stay with it. Change your thoughts! End your losing game!

Finally, after changing your behavior in the way you eat and the place you eat, and after dealing with emotional eating, add some suggestions to yourself to change the kind of food you eat to more healthful and nutritious foods, and put smaller portions on your plate.

A POWERFUL MOTIVATOR

If you have ever seen a loved one on a sick bed in a hospital or witnessed a person undergoing a heart attack, you can use these powerful negative associations as reminders every time you see a problem food that will make you fat and unhealthy.

See the person vividly, if you have had such an experience. Understand that poor health and bad eating and drinking habits lead to this condition.

YOUR NEW LIFE

Techniques in *TAPE IT OFF!* will work if you use them daily and will not work if you don't use them!

This may seem too obvious to mention, but I mention it anyway since you must understand that these relaxing daily fifteen minutes not only provide you with the new attitudes you will need to lose weight—they provide you with the emotional relaxation you need as well. *TAPE IT OFF!*, every day, for fifteen minutes!

Most people say they wouldn't give up this particular time anyway. It's too much fun! It relaxes you, and makes your evenings more enjoyable and refreshing. Many also use this technique in other facets of their lives beside eating and drinking. Some have used it to improve their golf and tennis games by "kicking in" positive images of themselves in a stressful time during the sports situation: that crucial serve in the final set, that nine-iron approach shot to the eighteenth green.

The body is a responsive biological creature, and it will respond to the person that knows it best—you!

WILL I NEED TO DO THIS FOREVER?

When you have reached your desired weight, you may find that it is possible to listen to your tape only three times a week, only on weeknights, or perhaps less. The answer to this question depends on your own personal characteristics.

You will have to gauge this yourself, watching your weight, and knowing that you can always *TAPE IT OFF!*

Now—go to it!

APPENDIX A

DESIRABLE WEIGHTS

A WORD OF ADVICE

Weigh yourself once a week at the same time of day, but *don't* put yourself through the daily grind of weighing and finding yourself depressed if you haven't lost any weight. With your new eating habits the pounds will come off steadily and regularly—but without the dizzying "yo-yo" effect you've experienced on crash "diets" that leave your body starved and crying out for nourishment. (Anxiety is the greatest mediating cause of overeating for many people, and daily weighing increases anxiety more often than not!) Friday morning is a good time to keep track of your progress on the scales.

HOW TO DETERMINE YOUR BODY FRAME BY ELBOW BREADTH

To make a simple approximation of your frame size:

Extend your arm and bend the forearm upwards at a 90 degree angle. Keep the fingers straight and turn the inside of your wrist away from the body. Place the thumb and index finger of your other

Source of basic data: *1979 Build Study,* Society of Actuaries and Association of Life Insurance Medical Directors of America, 1980. From the Metropolitan Life Insurance Company (used by permission).

1983 METROPOLITAN HEIGHT AND WEIGHT TABLE FOR MEN

Weights at Ages 25-59 Based on Lowest Mortality. Weight in Pounds According to Frame (in indoor clothing weighing 5 lbs., shoes with 1″ heels).

HEIGHT FEET	HEIGHT INCHES	SMALL FRAME	MEDIUM FRAME	LARGE FRAME
5	2	128-134	131-141	138-150
5	3	130-136	133-143	140-153
5	4	132-138	135-145	142-156
5	5	134-140	137-148	144-160
5	6	136-142	139-151	146-164
5	7	138-145	142-154	149-168
5	8	140-148	145-157	152-172
5	9	142-151	148-160	155-176
5	10	144-154	151-163	158-180
5	11	146-157	154-166	161-184
6	0	149-160	157-170	164-188
6	1	152-164	160-174	168-192
6	2	155-168	164-178	172-197
6	3	158-172	167-182	176-202
6	4	162-176	171-187	181-207

1983 METROPOLITAN HEIGHT AND WEIGHT TABLE FOR WOMEN

Weights at Ages 25-59 Based on Lowest Mortality. Weight in Pounds According to Frame (in indoor clothing weighing 3 lbs., shoes with 1″ heels).

HEIGHT FEET	HEIGHT INCHES	SMALL FRAME	MEDIUM FRAME	LARGE FRAME
4	10	102-111	109-121	118-131
4	11	103-113	111-123	120-134
5	0	104-115	113-126	122-137
5	1	106-118	115-129	125-140
5	2	108-121	118-132	128-143
5	3	111-124	121-135	131-147
5	4	114-127	124-138	134-151
5	5	117-130	127-141	137-155
5	6	120-133	130-144	140-159
5	7	123-136	133-147	143-163
5	8	126-139	136-150	146-167
5	9	129-142	139-153	149-170
5	10	132-145	142-156	152-173
5	11	135-148	145-159	155-176
6	0	138-151	148-162	158-179

hand on the two prominent bones on *either side* of your elbow. Measure the space between your fingers against a ruler or a tape measure.* Compare the measurements on the following tables.

These tables list the elbow measurements for medium-framed men and women of various heights. Measurements lower than those listed indicate you have a small frame and higher measurements indicate a large frame.

MEN

Height in 1″ heels	Elbow Breadth
5′2″–5′3″	2½″–2⅞″
5′4″–5′7″	2⅝″–2⅞″
5′8″–5′11″	2¾″–3″
6′0″–6′3″	2¾″–3⅛″
6′4″	2⅞″–3¼″

WOMEN

Height in 1″ heels	Elbow Breadth
4′10″–4′11″	2¼″–2½″
5′0″ –5′3″	2¼″–2½″
5′4″ –5′7″	2⅜″–2⅝″
5′8″ –5′11″	2⅜″–2⅝″
6′0″	2½″–2¾″

*For the most accurate measurement, have your physician measure your elbow breadth with a caliper.

APPENDIX B

SOME GOOD FOODS FOR YOUR SCRIPTS

In this section are listed some good foods and an eating philosophy to refresh your memory. But these are just reminders. You *know* what these foods are!

AN EATING (AND DRINKING) PHILOSOPHY

For many people, counting calories carefully focuses too much attention on eating. The rigor required to find the right foods for the "diet," correctly judge the size and weight of the portion, and find out the caloric impact of any unexpected preparation (breaded or sauced), plus recording in a diary—all of these raise your level of stress and tension, exactly the wrong way to approach food.

Taping it off will give you the relaxed attitude toward eating and drinking that you need. Just instruct yourself in your script to use these food groups at certain meals:

BREAKFAST
Fruit or small fruit juice
Cereal and skim milk
Tea or coffee

LUNCH
Chef's salad (or salad bar) with oil/vinegar or low-cal dressing
OR

Omelette (without high-calorie fillings or sauces!)
OR
Bread (or toast), 1 pat spread, 4 oz. cheese

DINNER
Tuna or turkey or chicken or fish or lean beef (4 oz.)
Cooked vegetables (2 of them, green and yellow)
A piece of bread or roll without spread

LATE SNACK (after a while you won't want one)
Diet gelatin or low-cal pudding (4 oz.)
OR
A blender shake (see below)

This is simple enough to remember without raising your anxiety feelings, and flexible enough to put some variety in your eating.

DRINKING

Your tape will relax you more effectively than the cocktail hour! True.

But those accustomed to cocktails retain skepticism on this point, so I suggest this: on your tape, give yourself the instruction that you will only enjoy cocktails on Friday and Saturday evenings. No lunchtimers. Don't worry about the amounts often given in "diets" (e.g. 1½ oz). Just limit yourself to Friday and Saturday evenings. Attempts to structure cocktail drinking, once started, are doubtful, since the essence of drinking is escape, release, relaxation, or inattention to detail.

Over a period of days you will see the evidence of the relaxing effect of your tape on Sunday through Thursday evenings. You may conclude then that a glass of wine with dinner will suffice!

One further suggestion: Try mixing a batch of cottage cheese with onion or bacon dip flavoring, and cutting up fresh vegetables to dip. Remember the times at a cocktail party when you said, "The dip and erudité hors d'oeuvres are enough for dinner by themselves!"

They can be! Make them Friday "dinner."

A WORD ABOUT BLENDERS

Blenders are useful tools for the weight-conscious, and come in inexpensive models. As thirst is often confused with hunger, you can deal with part of your "eating problem" by concocting low-calorie drinks—and blenders are excellent for this purpose.

Juice and skim-milk shakes can make satisfying substitutes for one or two meals a day, and nutritionist Richard A. Passwater provides a multitude of shake recipes in his book, *The Slendernow Diet* (St. Martin's Press/Richard Marek: 1982).

. . . AND ABOUT WATER

Drink more of it. An 8-ounce glass before meals, and in the evening snack period, will fill your stomach and help curb what you think is your appetite calling.

APPENDIX C

WEIGHT LOSS TABLE

The following table is for men and women, 36 to 55 years of age, between 5′6″ and 5′11″ in height. Figures for women are in italic type. The calorie-per-day figures of 900 for men and 2100 for women have not been calculated, as they are inappropriate for a gradual, steady weight-loss program. For complete tables covering different poundage losses, ages, and height levels, please see the book from which this table was derived. Adapted from *The Computer Diet* by Vincent Antonetti. (Copyright © 1973 by Vincent W. Antonetti. Reprinted by permission of the publisher, M. Evans and Company, Inc., New York, NY 10017.)

DAYS TO LOSE 40 POUNDS
(MEN: FROM 220 TO 180; WOMEN: FROM 180 TO 140)
(FIGURES FOR WOMEN ARE IN *ITALICS*.)

ACTIVITY LEVEL	CALORIES PER DAY 900	1200	1500	1800	2100
SEDENTARY (Inactive most of the day. Very little standing or walking.)	— *111*	100 *142*	124 *197*	164 *323*	242 —
LIGHT (Seated a major portion of the day. About 4 hours standing or walking. Typical of office work.)	— *103*	117 *129*	152 *172*	218 *261*	289 —
MODERATE (Stands as often as seated. Typical of teacher, young housewife, sales clerk.)	— *88*	98 *106*	122 *134*	160 *182*	236 —
VIGOROUS (Standing and walking most of day. Very little sitting. Typical of factory work, farmer, construction work.)	— *72*	78 *83*	93 *100*	113 *124*	146 —

APPENDIX D

EXERCISE AND ENERGY OUTPUT TABLES

This table shows the number of calories in some foods, and the minutes it would take a 150-pound person to use them up in various ways. (A 75-pound person would require twice as many minutes.) It should also show why you should use your tape to erase your desire for certain foods!

		MINUTES YOU WOULD NEED TO SPEND				
	CALORIES	LYING DOWN	WALKING	BICYCLE RIDING	SWIMMING	RUNNING
Banana, 7"	114	89	22	14	10	6
Beans (baked, w/brown sugar, 8-oz. can)	281	219	53	34	25	14
Beans (green, 1 cup)	30	23	6	4	3	1
Bread (8-oz. slice, Wonder cracked wheat)	60	47	11	7	5	3
Beer (11-oz. Michelob)	147	115	28	18	13	7
Egg (1 large, fried in butter)	99	78	19	12	9	5
Hamburger (Big-Mac, McDonald's)	561	438	107	67	50	28
Ice Cream (½ pint, Borden's, strawberry)	194	151	37	23	17	10

	CALORIES	MINUTES YOU WOULD NEED TO SPEND LYING DOWN	WALKING	BICYCLE RIDING	SWIMMING	RUNNING
Milkshake (McDonald's, chocolate)	318	248	60	38	29	16
Pie (Hostess, apple, 4½-oz.)	388	303	74	47	35	19
Pizza (Pizza Hut Supreme, ½ of 10″ pie)	475	371	90	57	43	24
Potato Salad (½ cup)	181	141	34	22	16	9
Spaghetti & meatballs (7½-oz. can)	222	173	42	27	20	11
Steak (Porterhouse, 16-oz. w/bone before cooking, lean & fat together)	1339	1044	254	161	121	67
lean only	372	290	71	45	33	19
Whiskey (2-oz. Southern Comfort, 86 proof)	168	131	32	20	15	8
Wine (4-oz. Beaujolais)	104	81	20	12	9	5

Adapted from Konishi, Frank: Food energy equivalents of various activities. Copyright The American Dietetic Association. Reprinted by permission from *Journal of the American Dietetic Association,* Vol. 46: 187, 1965. And from *The Barbara Kraus Brand Name Calorie Counter* (Avon, 1979). Used by permission.

INDEX